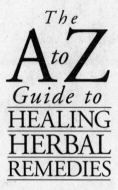

The
A to Z
Guide to
HEALING
HERBAL
REMEDIES

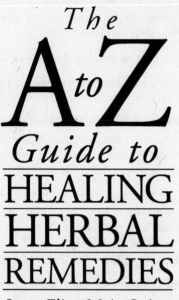

The
A to Z
Guide to
HEALING
HERBAL
REMEDIES

Jason Elias, M.A., L.Ac.,
and Shelagh Ryan Masline

A Lynn Sonberg Book

WINGS BOOKS
New York

Research about herbal remedies is ongoing and subject to interpretation. Although every effort has been made to include the most up-to-date and accurate information in this book, there can be no guarantee that what we know about this complex subject won't change with time. The reader should bear in mind that this book should not be used for self-diagnosis or self-treatment and should consult appropriate medical professionals regarding all health issues.

This 1997 edition is published by Wings Books,
a division of Random House Value Publishing, Inc.,
201 East 50th Street, New York, NY 10022,
by arrangement with Dell Publishing,
a division of Bantam Doubleday Dell Publishing Group, Inc.

Wings Books and colophon are trademarks of Random House Value Publishing, Inc.

Random House
New York • Toronto • London • Sydney • Auckland
http://www.randomhouse.com/

Printed and bound in the United States of America

Library of Congress Cataloging-in-Publication Data

Elias, Jason.
    The A to Z guide to healing herbal remedies / Jason Elias and Shelagh Ryan Masline.
        p.   cm.
    "A Lynn Sonberg book."
    Includes index.
    ISBN 0-517-14933-8
    1. Herbs—Therapeutic use—Encyclopedias.   I. Masline, Shelagh A. R.   II. Title
    RM666.H33E44   1997   96-36948
    615' .321—dc21   CIP

8 7 6 5 4 3 2 1

To Adam Benjamin Elias
and Caitlin Ryan Masline.
May all our children learn
of our innate potential to promote
the healing of our bodies
and our planet.

TABLE OF CONTENTS

Foreword xv
How to Use This Book xvii

PART ONE: Herbal Remedies for Optimum Health

Chapter 1. HEALING HERBS TODAY
Why You Need This Book 2
How Do We Know Herbs Work? 3
Rising Interest in Alternative Medicine 4
Theory of Herbal Medicine 5
    A Holistic Approach 6
    Where Disease Comes From 6
Prevention Is the Key 8
Herbs for Ailments 10

Chapter 2. USING HERBAL REMEDIES
A Variety of Herbal Preparations 12
Safety Guidelines When Using Herbs 18
How to Find a Qualified Herbalist 20
Where to Purchase Herbal Remedies 21
Mail Order Sources of Herbs 22

Chapter 3. HERBS FOR OPTIMUM HEALTH AND
          VITALITY
The Changing Face of Disease 25
What Are Herbal Tonics? 27
Get Heart-Smart 28

Boost Your Immune System.............................. 30
Improve Your Digestion................................ 32
Get Rid of the Toxins in Your Body.................... 34
Breathe Easy 36
Nourish Your Reproductive System and
    Add Sexual Vigor.................................. 38
Get on Top of Stress 40
Look Your Best 42

PART TWO: Healing Herbs: An A to Z Guide

AGNUS-CASTUS (*Vitex agnus-castus*) 47
AGRIMONY (*Agrimonia eupatoria*)...................... 48
ALFALFA (*Medicago sativa*) 50
ALMOND (*Prunus amygdalus*) 51
ALOE VERA (*Aloe barbadenis*) 53
ANGELICA (*Angelica archangelica*) 55
ANISEED (*Pimpinella anisum*)......................... 56
ARNICA (*Arnica montana*)............................. 58
ARTICHOKE (*Cynara scolymus*) 59
ASPARAGUS ROOT (*Asparagus officinalis*) 60
ASTRAGALUS (*Astragalus membranaceous*) 62
BALM OF GILEAD (*Populus gileadensis*) 64
BARBERRY (*Berberis vulgaris*)........................ 65
BAYBERRY (*Myrica cerifera*).......................... 66
BISTORT (*Polygonum bistorta*) 68
BLACK COHOSH (*Cimicifuga racemosa*).................. 69
BLACK HAW (*Viburnum prunifolium*).................... 71
BLESSED THISTLE (*Cnicus benedictus*) 73
BONESET (*Eupatorium perfoliatum*).................... 74
BUCHU (*Barosma betulina or Agathosma betulina*) ... 76
BURDOCK (*Arctium lappa*) 77
BUTCHER'S-BROOM (*Ruscus aculeatus*) 79

CALENDULA (*Calendula officinalis*) 80

CASCARA SAGRADA (*Rhamnus purshiana*) 82

CATNIP (*Nepeta cataria*) 83

CAYENNE (*Capsicum frutescens*) 85

CHAMOMILE (*Matricaria chamomilla*) 87

CHAPARRAL (*Larrea tridentata*)........................ 89

CLEAVERS (*Galium aparine*)............................. 91

CLOVES (*Caryophyllus aromaticus*)...................... 93

COLTSFOOT (*Tussilago farfara*)......................... 94

COMFREY (*Symphytum officinale*) 97

CRAMP BARK (*Viburnum opulus*)....................... 99

CRANBERRY (*Vaccinium macrocarpon*) 101

CRANESBILL (*Geranium maculatum*).................. 102

DAMIANA (*Turnera aphrodisiaca or diffusa*).......... 103

DANDELION (*Taraxacum officinale*)................... 105

DEVIL'S-CLAW (*Harpagophytum procumbens*) 107

DILL (*Anethum graveolens*)............................... 108

DONG QUAI (*Angelica senensis*)........................ 110

ECHINACEA (*Echinacea angustifolia*)................. 111

ELDER (*Sambucus nigra*)................................. 114

ELECAMPANE (*Inula helenium*) 115

EPHEDRA (*Ephedra sinica*)............................. 116

EUCALYPTUS (*Eucalyptus globulus*)................... 119

EVENING PRIMROSE (*Oenothera biennis*) 121

EYEBRIGHT (*Euphrasia officinalis*) 122

FALSE UNICORN ROOT (*Chamaelirium luteum*) 123

FENNEL (*Foeniculum vulgare*)........................... 125

FENUGREEK (*Trigonella foenumgraecum*)............. 126

FEVERFEW (*Tanacetum parthenium*) 128

FO-TI (*Polygonum multiflorum*) 130

GARLIC (*Allium sativum*) 131

GENTIAN (*Gentiana lutea*)............................... 134

GINGER (*Zingiber officinale*) 136

GINKGO (*Ginkgo biloba*)............................138

GINSENG, AMERICAN (*Panax quinquefolium*).......140

GINSENG, ASIAN (*Panax ginseng*)....................143

GINSENG, SIBERIAN (*Eleutherococcus senticosus*) 145

GOAT'S RUE (*Galega officinalis*)......................148

GOLDENSEAL (*Hydrastis canadensis*) 149

GOTU KOLA (*Centella asiatica*) 151

HAWTHORN (*Crataegus oxyacantha*) 153

HOPS (*Humulus lupulus*)................................155

HORSE CHESTNUT (*Aesculus hippocastanum*).......156

HORSETAIL (*Equisetum arvense*) 157

JUNIPER (*Juniperus communis*) 159

LADY'S MANTLE (*Alchemilla vulgaris* and *xanthochlora*)..161

LAVENDER (*Lavandula officinalis*) 162

LEMON BALM (*Melissa officinalis*) 163

LICORICE (*Glycyrrhiza glabra*) 165

LOBELIA (*Lobelia inflata*) 167

MARIGOLD (*Calendula officinalis*) 170

MEADOWSWEET (*Filipendula ulmaria* or *Spiraea ulmaria*)..171

MILK THISTLE (*Silybum marianum*)...................173

MOTHERWORT (*Leonurus cardiaca*) 175

MULLEIN (*Verbascum thapsus*)..........................176

MYRRH (*Commiphora myrrha*)..........................178

OATS (*Avena sativa*)......................................180

PAPAYA (*Carica papaya*) 181

PARSLEY (*Petroselinum sativum*) 183

PAU D'ARCO (*Tabebuia heptaphylla*)..................184

PEPPERMINT (*Mentha piperita*) 185

PLANTAIN *(Plantago major)* 187
PSYLLIUM *(Plantago psyllium)* 188
RASPBERRY *(Rubus idaeus)*............................190
RED CLOVER *(Trifolium pratense)* 191
ROSEMARY *(Rosmarinus officinalis)* 193
ST. JOHN'S WORT *(Hypericum perforatum)* 194
SAW PALMETTO *(Serenoa serrulata)* 196
SLIPPERY ELM *(Ulmus rubra)*........................198
THYME *(Thymus vulgaris)* 199
UVA-URSI *(Arctostaphylos uva-ursi)*....................201
VALERIAN *(Valeriana officinalis)* 203
VERVAIN *(Verbena officinalis)*...........................204
WHITE WILLOW *(Salix alba)*...........................206
WILD CHERRY BARK *(Prunus serotina)*..............208
WILD INDIGO *(Baptisia tinctoria)*......................209
WITCH HAZEL *(Hamamelis virginiana)* 210
WOOD BETONY *(Betonica officinalis)* 211
YARROW *(Achillea millefolium)* 212
YELLOW DOCK *(Rumex crispus)*....................214

PART THREE: Herbal Combinations for Symptoms and Ailments

Symptoms and Ailments: Which Herbal
  Remedy Is Right for You?...........................219
An Herbal Combination for What Ails You..........219
ACNE...221
AIDS (Acquired Immune Deficiency Syndrome).......222
ARTHRITIS..223
ASTHMA 224
ATHLETE'S FOOT 225
BAD BREATH 226
BRONCHITIS 227

BRUISES 228
BURNS 229
CANCER 229
CHOLESTEROL, HIGH LEVELS 230
CHRONIC FATIGUE 231
CIRRHOSIS...232
COLDS 233
COLD SORES 234
COLIC 235
CONJUNCTIVITIS 236
CONSTIPATION 237
COUGHS...238
DEPRESSION 240
DIABETES MELLITUS................................241
DIARRHEA 242
DIGESTIVE PROBLEMS............................243
DIZZINESS 244
EAR PROBLEMS 245
EMPHYSEMA...246
FEVER 246
FLATULENCE (Gas) 248
FLU 249
FOOD POISONING 250
HAIR LOSS...250
HAY FEVER...251
HEADACHE 252
HEART PROBLEMS 253
HEMORRHOIDS.......................................253
HEPATITIS..254
HERPES SIMPLEX....................................255
HYPERTENSION 256
INDIGESTION 256

INFERTILITY 257
INSOMNIA 259
LIVER PROBLEMS 259
MENOPAUSE 260
MENSTRUAL PROBLEMS 261
MOTION SICKNESS 263
NAUSEA 263
PAIN 264
PALPITATIONS 265
POISON IVY 266
PMS (Premenstrual Syndrome) 267
PROSTATE PROBLEMS 267
PSORIASIS 268
SORE THROAT 269
STRESS 269
SUNBURN 271
TOOTH AND GUM PROBLEMS 271
URINARY-TRACT INFECTIONS 272
VARICOSE VEINS 273
WHOOPING COUGH 274
WOUNDS 274
YEAST INFECTIONS 275

Index 277
About the Authors 293

FOREWORD

Your body, an amazing work of art, has an innate intelligence that is more complicated than the most sophisticated computer. Every day your body creates and destroys hundreds of cancer cells, any one of which, if it escaped the vigilance of your immune system, could lead to serious illness. Two years from now all the cells in your body will be different; this, to me, is miraculous.

When a person walks into my office, it is never just a symptom I greet—I welcome a human being as rich as a tapestry, unique in his or her experiences and way of being in the world. I see symptoms as manifestations of a lack of harmony, either within a person or in the person's relationship to the world. My concept of healing is to assist my clients in restoring that harmony.

The Chinese have an analogy: to treat a diseased tree by simply cutting off its symptomatic branch will send the disease deeper. For every afflicted branch cut, two more will erupt. We can effectively cut the branch only if we also treat the root.

A good herbal prescription will include herbs that can alleviate symptoms and ailments (lack of appetite, headache, painful joints, lower back pain, premenstrual cramps, and so forth)—but it will also have herbs that support you as an individual and enable you to tap into your own magnificent healing resources. The word *healing* comes from the same root as *wholeness* does—herbs will help you to heal yourself and be whole once more.

In this book you will find that herbalism is a natural way to supplement conventional medical care. If you are fed up with the anonymity and depersonalization of traditional Western medicine, herbalism is a viable alternative that respects your humanity and gives you personal responsibility for your own health.

The beauty of herbs lies in their ability to help your own body/mind heal itself, a process that it naturally does most efficiently. As Voltaire said, "The art of medicine consists of amusing the patient while nature cures the disease." The biggest gift I can give you is the knowledge that you have the power to heal yourself. And the very real joy I experience in treating my clients is seeing them gradually feeling better and taking more control of themselves, in body, mind, and spirit.

Jason Elias, M.A., L.Ac.

HOW TO USE THIS BOOK

In *Healing Herbal Remedies* you will have an opportunity to acquaint yourself with the many different varieties of herbs, to gather information on how to use herbal remedies safely and effectively, and to learn how herbs act on your body's systems and organs. Our first three chapters, Part I, provide you with a sound introduction to herbalism and the various ways herbs are used as tonics and to treat certain conditions and ailments.

In Part II of this book, "Healing Herbs: An A to Z Guide," we will introduce you to over one hundred herbs. You will see that each has its own individual personality and set of healing actions. Some herbs are powerful; others are gentle. There are restorative tonics for the elderly and herbs mild yet effective enough to ease your baby's colic. There are herbs for men and herbs for women. Take your time and get acquainted with these herbs.

This section is organized alphabetically according to the name of each herb. It is extremely easy to use. Each entry includes:

▼ A general description of the herb
▼ Which parts of the herb are used
▼ The primary function of the herb
▼ Other benefits that the herb may offer
▼ Recommended preparations and dosages

▼ Any general or special precautions you should take while using this herbal remedy

Take particular note of special precautions; certain herbs require special care if, for example, you are pregnant or suffering from a prior medical condition.

Turn to Part III to find information about how to treat specific symptoms and ailments with herbal combinations. Like Part II, this section is arranged in alphabetical order for easy reference. We describe the nature of each condition and suggest herbs that are particularly appropriate for dealing with your problem. Remember that herbs are synergistic; a combination of herbs is usually greater—that is, more effective—than the sum of its parts.

It's important to remember here that it's not a good idea to try mixing and matching herbs yourself. It takes years of training and clinical experience to acquire the expertise to do this. If, on the other hand, you want to treat a simple ailment yourself, you can try the herbal combination we recommend in this section. Alternatively, you may choose from a variety of commercial formulas, readily available in health food stores and herb shops, in which various herbs are already combined.

You can also take a single herb as a remedy. For example, choose raw garlic mixed with honey or on a piece of bread to treat a sore throat; take ginger to relieve a mild case of nausea or seasickness; valerian is a good relaxant; and many people choose echinacea as an immune tonic. These are all generally safe bets.

Of course, if you are taking other medications or have a specific medical condition, remember to consult an herbalist or herbally oriented physician before trying herbal remedies. Always pay close attention to the proper use of each herbal remedy. And keep in mind that herbs are meant to supplement—not replace—traditional medical care when dealing with serious illness.

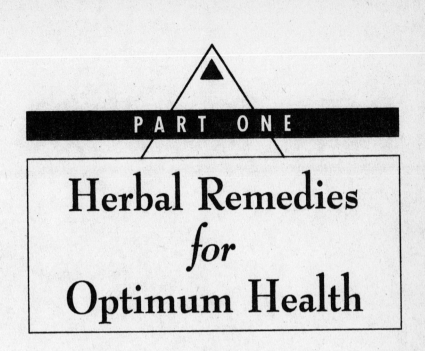

PART ONE

Herbal Remedies
for
Optimum Health

CHAPTER 1
Healing Herbs Today

Herbs have an enormous and exciting range of healing powers. The use of herbs—remedies prepared from roots, leaves, and other parts of plants—is an age-old way in which you can both increase your overall resistance to disease and hasten your recovery from all types of illnesses. Modern health experts are putting more and more emphasis on the first part of that equation—promoting health and preventing disease. Don't wait until you get sick; herbal tonics can help you stay well.

Hawthorn, for example, nurtures and supports your heart. Elecampane is one of the most effective herbal strengtheners of the respiratory system. And there's a very special herb called gentian that you can carry with you when you travel: a drop on the tongue before eating a meal in a foreign country can save you from a bout with that notorious "friend" of travelers, diarrhea.

Of course, you can also reach for herbal remedies when you do get sick. Herbs alleviate a wide range of symptoms and ailments, from the simplest to the most profound. Try a drop of clove or myrrh tincture to ease toothache pain. If you're the nursing mom of a colicky baby, sip a cup of mild chamomile tea. Passing this soothing remedy on through breast milk might just relieve your baby's discomfort—and help you get a good night's sleep.

Herbs can also be a valuable addition to the regular

1

medical care of very serious and even life-threatening diseases. An excellent Chinese tonic called astragalus can enhance your immune system. So can echinacea and red clover, both often enlisted by herbalists in the war against cancer and AIDS. And while neither drug nor herb can reverse the destruction of cirrhosis, liver tonics such as dandelion and milk thistle can help prevent further damage.

In short, herbal remedies can play a key role in supporting your overall health. Every day new scientific studies emerge proving the validity of traditional herbal remedies. We now know that herbal remedies can be a safe, natural, and accessible alternative to synthetic drugs. Moreover, herbs are less expensive and have fewer side effects than conventional drugs. In this book you'll learn how to stay healthy the safe and natural way.

Why You Need This Book

Perhaps you picked up this book already convinced of the healing power of herbs. But does this mean that you can simply stroll over to your local health food store or herb shop and pick out an herbal remedy for painful menstrual cramps or constipation? Unfortunately, it's not so easy.

The reason you need this book is that you will find very little useful information on the labels of herbal remedies in your health food store, herb shop, or supermarket. Why is that? The approval process of the United States Food and Drug Administration has caused us to lag far behind other countries in the use and regulation of herbs. An herb, unlike a drug, cannot be patented by any one company in the United States—which means that manufacturers of these remedies have little incentive to brave the costly and lengthy gauntlet of the FDA's approval process.

In consequence, most healing herbs are not approved by the FDA; therefore, the FDA cannot allow the packagers of herbal products to make any healing claims on the labels of their products. Even more significantly, and potentially more harmful to consumers, the FDA does not permit warning of any possible side effects of herbs.

We enter the health store or herb shop in a quandary. Legally, there can be little information of value on the labels of herbal remedies. Just what will these garlic capsules do for me? I have a migraine; which of these remedies can give me some relief? I've heard that aloe is a good remedy for sunburn, but it's a hot summer day and they're all sold out; is there another natural remedy for sunburn?

You won't find the answers to these questions on the labels of herbal remedies, but you will find them in this book. Carry this book with you to the health food store or herb shop—our clear and simple organization will enable you to choose the herbal remedy that is right for you.

How Do We Know Herbs Work?

Long before there was such a thing as a doctor, people were using herbs for medicinal purposes. And, over the years, our ancestors discovered by trial and error which plants had healing properties and which were poisonous.

You may be surprised to learn that up until this century most medicines used in the United States were herbal. But when wonder drugs such as penicillin were discovered in the 1920s, the popularity of herbal remedies began to wane in the United States. Ironically, during the period that traditional herbal remedies were frowned upon, modern medicine co-opted their use. A large percentage—up to 25 percent of modern prescription and over-the-counter drugs—are actually derived from herbs.

Herbal remedies have never lost their enormous popularity in Europe. In countries such as England, France, and Germany, where scientific studies are regularly conducted on herbs, evidence that supports and even expands the range of healing abilities of herbs emerges on a regular basis. In fact, herbs and more conventional medicines stand side by side on the pharmacy shelves of Europe, and it is not unusual for doctors to recommend an herbal remedy rather than prescribing a drug for their patients.

Rising Interest in Alternative Medicine

Over the last twenty years there has been a dramatic resurgence of interest in herbal remedies in the United States. As scientific evidence mounts in support of herbalism and other alternative forms of treatment, experts predict that American medicine is poised for dramatic change. In 1992 the National Institutes of Health (NIH) established an Office of Alternative Medicine to explore the potential benefits of herbal remedies and other alternatives to conventional medical care. Medical schools are also coming around: even Harvard Medical School is joining the ranks of institutions offering courses on so-called unorthodox medicine.

A January 1993 study in *The New England Journal of Medicine* reported that 34 percent of all Americans have used some form of alternative medicine. Clearly, Americans are seeking a more humane and less invasive approach than that of standard medical doctors. According to Dr. Joe Jacobs, director of the NIH Office of Alternative Medicine, "Some of these alternative therapies take a holistic and more caring view of a patient." This holistic attitude is an important foundation of the theory of herbalism, one that we'll soon explore more fully.

Herbal remedies are not intended to replace mainstream medical care. But healing herbal remedies are indeed a precious addition to regular medical care—one that we unfortunately lost sight of for some time this century, and have rediscovered at a critical juncture in the American health care system.

Theory of Herbal Medicine

The goal of herbalism is to help you keep yourself well. The herbal way enables you take charge of your own well-being on every level: mentally, spiritually, emotionally, and physically. Our approach empowers you to mobilize your body's own natural defenses to stay healthy.

When illness strikes, herbal remedies act differently on our bodies than conventional medicines. While conventional medicines are designed to cure the symptoms of a specific disease or ailment, herbal treatments enable you to activate your own resources to combat the hostile bacterial or viral invaders—what herbalists call the underlying toxic state—that are causing your symptoms.

Many herbalists actually see the standard medical practice of suppressing symptoms as an interruption of your body's natural healing processes. Symptoms such as diarrhea, vomiting, coughing, and headaches are your body's natural way of cleansing itself of toxins. But you don't just have to suffer through them—many herbal remedies also act to ease the discomfort you feel while your body purges itself of the underlying toxins.

A Holistic Approach

Herbal medicine, like most other forms of alternative medicine, takes a holistic approach to healing. This means viewing the patient as a whole person while emphasizing health and wellness and the prevention of disease. To an herbalist, you are much more than an interesting set of symptoms that must be somehow eradicated with the proper medicine. You are a complex human being, functioning on mental, spiritual, and emotional as well as physical levels.

In this book you will learn that you are in charge of keeping your body well. One of the first ways to prevent disease is to embrace a healthy lifestyle. Read on as we explore some of the negative factors that may cause disease. Do you incorporate any of them into your own lifestyle? If so, you have the knowledge and the strength to change them.

Where Disease Comes From

Herbal practitioners believe that a primary cause of disease is the presence of unhealthy elements in your lifestyle. A poor diet, too much stress, lack of exercise, and uneducated behavior such as smoking put your body in what herbalists call a state of toxemia. The important thing to remember is that you are in control—these are all habits that you yourself have the power to change.

Modern medicine is actually not so far off in its current explanation of where disease comes from. Scientific studies abound linking diets high in fat to heart disease and cancer, high levels of stress and anger to increased risk of heart attacks, and smoking to lung cancer. But a major difference is that modern medicine, in contrast to herbalism and other alternative approaches, continues to focus on alleviating symptoms rather than preventing disease.

Where Do Headaches Come From?

Let's take a look at one symptom: a headache. A simple headache can be caused by a wide range of underlying conditions, such as digestive disorders, muscular tension, PMS, stress, or eyestrain.

To simply relieve headache pain doesn't deal with where that headache is coming from. If your headache is the result, for example, of constipation, you may require a digestive aid as well as relief from the pain of the headache.

Try to identify and treat the underlying condition that has led to your headache. Perhaps it is stress. What is the source of your stress? Can you remove it? If not, there are many routes you can take: a brisk walk and a cup of valerian tea might just do the trick, restoring your body to its normal balance, strength, and vitality.

If headaches persist and you cannot identify and relieve their underlying cause, your best bet is to visit a qualified professional who can help you do so.

Prevention Is the Key

Let's take a look at prevention and lifestyle—this is what herbalism is really all about. Herbal medicine goes hand in hand with the preventive methods that are gaining in popularity every day. Let's again focus our attention on a holistic approach to your health, on leading a healthy lifestyle rather than on relieving symptoms. It's time to take responsibility for our own health rather than wait for symptoms to occur and then treat them. In this way we will all lead healthier lives. We will seize control of our health, and prevention will come to replace intervention.

The most up-to-date medical data clearly relate your level of physical and mental well-being with your lifestyle. Your diet, emotions, exercise, and other behavior patterns all affect your vulnerability to disease. Improper diet is an important factor in causing heart problems, cancer, and other diseases. Living under a high level of stress can lead to an attack of hives—and it can also put you at greater risk for certain forms of cancer. Regular exercise is good for both our bodies and our minds. And unwise habits—such as smoking cigarettes or drinking too many cocktails—should be avoided. They increase our risk of many types of serious disease, including heart problems and cancer

The typical American diet is too high in fat, processed foods, and meat, and too low in whole grains and fiber-rich fruits and vegetables. Studies show that high-fat diets increase your risk of developing breast, prostate, and colon cancer. On the other hand, a high-fiber diet can reduce your risk of colon cancer, and eating lots of vitamin-packed fruits, vegetables, and whole grains can reduce your risk for a wide range of diseases. Use the principles of good nutrition to come up with ways in which you can improve your own diet.

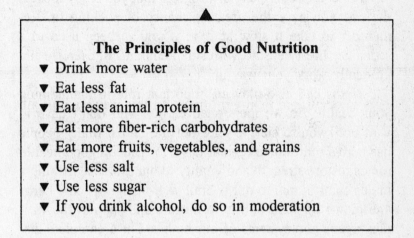

The Principles of Good Nutrition

▼ Drink more water
▼ Eat less fat
▼ Eat less animal protein
▼ Eat more fiber-rich carbohydrates
▼ Eat more fruits, vegetables, and grains
▼ Use less salt
▼ Use less sugar
▼ If you drink alcohol, do so in moderation

Your emotions also affect your susceptibility to disease. Tension and anxiety, worries and fears—these stressful conditions not only have impact on our psyches, we now know that they also have dangerous, and sometimes fatal, implications for our bodily health. What is stress? Anything that creates a physical state of arousal that prepares you to face whatever challenge is at hand. The stimuli that lead to stress can be physical or emotional. They range from important life events, such as a death in the family or a divorce, to day-to-day hassles, like dealing with rush-hour traffic.

Regular exercise is one very important way to reduce stress in your life. In fact, exercise is a vital key to your overall good health. Twenty minutes each day of your favorite aerobic exercise—such as walking, biking, or swimming —not only eases stress, it also strengthens your heart and lungs, gets your circulation going, and helps you sleep better. The exercise or exercise program that you enjoy most is the one you have the greatest chance of sticking to. Remember to take it slow at first: if you've been used to a sedentary lifestyle, start with small amounts of exercise and gradually work your way up.

Herbs can also play an important role in maintaining your health. As we mentioned earlier, you don't have to wait until you're sick to take out the herbs. Many people use herbal tonics on a regular basis for general good health: tonics restore strength and vitality to our systems, making a major contribution to our overall well-being. Specific herbs are known for their ability to nurture and support the various organs and systems of our bodies. For a complete discussion of the use of herbs to promote health and prevent disease, turn to Chapter Three.

Herbs for Ailments

Despite all the precautions we take and regardless of how carefully we lead our healthy lifestyles, sometimes we just get sick. Experiencing an ailment means that your body is trying to purge excess poisons from your system. As you fight off a virus or bacteria, you may experience a wide range of symptoms, such as diarrhea or constipation, headaches, body aches and pains, lethargy, vomiting, sweating, skin rashes, and excessive discharge of mucus.

Remember that these symptoms—uncomfortable as they may seem at the time—are a positive action on your body's part to rid itself of excess toxins. Appropriate herbal remedies will help your body solve the underlying problem that has caused your symptoms. Herbs can hasten the healing process, and ease any discomfort you may experience while you are getting better.

When the ailment is a minor one that you can treat at home, reach for *Healing Herbal Remedies* to see which herbal medicine is the best for you. Minor ailments will naturally respond to herbal treatment more quickly than serious diseases. Ginger is often a quick remedy for motion sickness and nausea; aniseed is an excellent remedy for flatulence; and aloe vera can relieve painful sunburn.

If you suffer from a serious disease, talk to your medical doctor about supplementing your regular treatment with visits to a qualified herbalist, or find a medical doctor who also practices alternative medicine. While most health professionals believe that it is not appropriate to use herbal remedies alone to treat critical diseases such as cancer, modern medical researchers are discovering that many herbs—such as chaparral and red clover—show promising anticancer action.

In each individual case, however, it is the nature of the ailment that will determine how long it is appropriate to use an herbal remedy. If a minor condition does not respond to herbal treatment in two or three weeks, it is time for professional consultation. Serious diseases, again, require professional attention. For complete information on the safe use of herbs, see page 18.

CHAPTER 2
Using Herbal Remedies

Now that you have begun to understand the herbal approach to good health, it's time to learn how safe and easy it is to incorporate herbs into your everyday lifestyle. A virtual cornucopia of good health awaits you in a wide variety of herbal forms. You can purchase dried herbs in many health food stores and herb shops, and you can make your own remedies. You can visit a qualified herbalist. Or you can take advantage of the many commercially prepared herbal remedies lined up on the shelves of your local store.

In this chapter we'll describe the different types of herbal remedies, and offer some hints on how to best use each one. Remember that it's important to practice basic safety guidelines when taking any remedy. We'll also take a look at how to locate a qualified herbal practitioner, and where it's best to purchase herbal remedies.

A Variety of Herbal Preparations

The many methods of preparing herbal remedies have developed through trial and error over the course of centuries, as herbalists have found that each individual herb releases its healing powers most effectively in certain forms. The constituents of some herbs are most productively activated when they are prepared as decoctions, while in the case of other herbs, capsules prove to be a more appropriate choice. In this book you can look under the alphabetical listing of each herbal remedy to review the preparations and dosages that are most appropriate for that herb's unique blend of healing actions.

You may not be acquainted with words like *decoctions* and *infusions,* but once you read about them you'll find that they're not nearly so daunting as they may at first appear. In fact, if you know how to make a cup of tea, it is certain that you will be able to produce both. Here we define the various types of herbal remedies for the reader in plain, straightforward language. We also offer a few practical tips on how you yourself can make them. If you want to make your own herbal remedy, it's best to do so as a decoction or an infusion.

Decoction   A decoction is a remedy made by boiling the hard and woody parts of herbs. Break up the bark or roots into small pieces—the smaller they are, the more easily they'll be absorbed into the water. A great deal of heat is necessary to make sure that the active constituents of the herb—those healing juices that have a specific dynamic effect on your body—are released. More heat is needed in making decoctions than infusions, since the parts of the herb that are used in decoctions—the bark and roots—are very dense in nature.

To make a decoction, boil 1 ounce of the herb in 4 cups of water. Allow the water to boil for about 10 minutes, until it has been reduced to approximately 3 cups. Next, add any lighter material, such as the flowers and leaves you would use to make infusions. Cover and steep for an additional 10 minutes, and then strain the mixture.

Decoctions will last three or four days in the refrigerator. In this book, the dosages of decoctions are usually given in cups per day. A note of caution here: If you are using a combination of herbs in a decoction or infusion, use 1 ounce of the *total* combined herbs recommended—*not* 1 ounce of each single herb. Use stainless steel or ceramic pots to make herbal remedies; avoid using aluminum, which may chemically interact with the mixtures.

Infusion   An infusion is another easy way to make an herbal remedy. Again the goal is to extract the active qualities, or healing juices, of the herb. Start by bruising 1 ounce of dried flowers, leaves, or petals of the herb in a clean cloth. Then pour 3 cups of boiling water over the herb. Cover the mixture closely and let it steep for 20 to 30 minutes. Strain the mixture, and drink it hot or cold.

Like decoctions, infusions should be refrigerated and generally last three or four days. Dosages of infusions are also given in cups per day. And again take note: If you are using a combination of herbs in a decoction or infusion, use 1 ounce of the *total* combined herbs recommended—*not* 1 ounce of each single herb.

Tincture   Professional herbalists often prepare tinctures especially designed to meet the unique needs of their patients. More broad-based commercial tinctures are available in health food stores and herb shops. Tinctures are strong preparations that should be stored in cool places and out of the reach of children.

In tinctures we use alcohol to extract the active qualities of the herb. Because tinctures are much more potent than decoctions or infusions, dosages are given in smaller amounts. In this book we recommend tinctures in terms of teaspoons per day. If you use a commercial remedy, dosages may also be given in drops or milliliters; carefully follow the directions on each remedy.

A tincture is made by pouring 5 ounces of alcohol over

1 ounce of a dried herb or 3 ounces of fresh herbs. Many commercial tinctures are made from pure grain alcohol (198 proof); others use a combination of alcohol and water. Shake tinctures twice each day to maintain their blend of active ingredients.

Most people prefer to get tinctures from a qualified herbal practitioner or from a reputable company. But if you want to make your own at home, here's how you go about it: Combine 5 ounces of 100 proof vodka and 1 ounce of the herb in a small, sterile, airtight bottle. Over time the active qualities of the herb are released into the alcohol. Tinctures require 2 to 6 weeks to make, but they can last over a year.

For those who don't care for alcohol, you can use vinegar instead of vodka. Or add the tincture to 1 cup of warm water—this will cause most of the alcohol to evaporate, as well as diluting any bitter taste.

Tea Herbal teas are very pleasant, but they do not have medicinal dosages of the active constituents of herbs. Still, they do have a mild relaxing or invigorating effect, according to the character of the herb used to make the tea. Herbal teas can also be a healthy addition to your daily diet; try substituting herbal teas for caffeine-laden coffee or sugary sodas.

▲

How to Make a Medicinal Cup of Tea

A useful shortcut to making a decoction or infusion is to take 3 herbal tea bags (triple the usual amount) and steep them in 1 covered cup of very hot

water for 10 minutes. Voilà! By tripling the amount
of the herb used, you have extracted many more of its
active constituents. You have achieved a very reason-
able equivalent of a potent herbal remedy—a decoction or infusion.

Extract Commercial extracts are, like tinctures,
available in health food stores and herb shops. Some professional herbalists also prepare extracts. Extracts are con-
centrated extractions of fresh herbs, but the medium used in
extracts—unlike in tinctures—is water rather than alcohol.
Since alcohol is a preservative, tinctures tend to last much
longer than extracts. Refrigerated extracts, which are usually mixed in water or juice, last only about a week. Store-
bought extracts may last longer because they usually include glycerine or alcohol.

Capsules and Pills Capsules and pills contain dried
herbs. Unlike liquid remedies, no extraction process has
been used in their preparation. Capsules and pills can be a
great convenience when you're on the go—whether simply
in the course of your normal day, or when you're traveling
for pleasure or off on a business trip.

Some herbalists believe, however, that capsules and
pills have certain disadvantages compared to liquid-based
internal remedies. While capsules may be preferable in certain conditions, such as when you want the herbs released
in the intestines rather than the stomach, liquid remedies
are generally better, for a number of reasons. First, the active constituents of the herbs are not as readily available to
your body when they are in capsule or pill form. Heat and

water in the processes we describe above help release the healing agents of herbs; digestion alone does not guarantee that this takes place.

Second, many people prefer capsules because some herbs taste bitter. The problem here is that experiencing the bitter taste itself is important in order to receive the full benefits of the herb. The bitter taste is what provokes an important series of bodily actions, such as stimulating bile flow and digestive juices, regulating insulin, releasing the hormone gastrin, and more. These functions are useful in the treatment of digestive disorders, diabetes, gall bladder problems, liver disease, and other ailments.

Still, many herbalists continue to recommend herbal capsules and pills, and they are certainly very handy in today's busy and active world. Capsules, by the way, can also be opened and the powder inside them can be made into infusions or decoctions. And chewing rather than swallowing pills can help release their vital constituents.

The dosages of pills and capsules vary widely. Capsules come in different sizes. Carefully follow the directions on the bottle of any commercial herbal remedy you choose, beginning your usage with the smallest recommended dose.

Mouthwash Many herbal mouthwashes can be used to reduce tooth decay and relieve sore gums or throats. Myrrh is especially good for mouth and gum infections. Gargling with bayberry mouthwash can relieve sore throats and gums. You can usually use mouthwash up to three times daily.

Douche An herbal douche is a liquid remedy inserted into a body cavity for cleansing or curative reasons. Vaginal douches are most common. For example, a douche made with echinacea and pau d'arco can be used three times a week for the duration of a yeast infection. Herbal douches are available commercially and from herbalists. In general, douches should not be used too often. If the condition you are treating with a douche persists, consult a qualified practitioner.

Compress   A hot compress may be made by pouring a hot herbal tea on a towel. (Be careful that the tea is not so hot it burns you.) Many compresses are helpful in relieving swollen conditions. Apply compresses locally as needed.

Poultice   Poultices are hot packs applied to the skin to help heal a wound. To make a poultice, mix the ground herb with hot water. Put the mixture into a muslin bag and apply to the affected area as needed.

Cream, Oil, Ointment, Salve   These often have an herbal basis and can be applied locally as needed. They can promote the healing of and be very soothing to burns and superficial wounds. Carefully follow the instructions on the label of a commercial remedy, and begin use with the lowest recommended dosage. Discontinue treatment if you develop any sort of rash.

Safety Guidelines When Using Herbs

As we have seen, herbal remedies are a safe and natural way to keep your body strong and healthy and to help prevent and heal disease. Yet herbs have potent actions on your body, and naturally precautions should be taken when using any herbal remedy.

Every herbal profile in this book includes a section on precautions. "General Precautions" indicate that you should simply exercise good common sense in the use of this remedy as with any other. When "Special Precautions" should be taken with an herb (for example, if an herb should be strictly avoided during pregnancy or if you suffer from a chronic condition such as diabetes), we spell out these precautions in careful detail.

Here are a few general safety tips to keep in mind when using herbal remedies:

▼ Pregnant and nursing women should consult with their obstetrician, midwife, or herbally oriented practitioner before using medicinal amounts of any herb.

▼ Herbal remedies are generally not appropriate for children under two. Sit down with your pediatrician and discuss the situation before administering any herb to infants or toddlers.

▼ People have different sensitivity levels to medication. It is good common sense to begin with lowest recommended dosages of remedies, and increase gradually as needed.

▼ Herbal remedies should be used with caution by those over sixty-five. Elderly people should be especially careful to begin and perhaps remain with the lowest recommended dosages of herbal preparations.

▼ If you suffer from a chronic illness, confer with a qualified herbal professional or an herbally trained physician before taking an herbal remedy.

▼ Herbs can interact with prescription and over-the-counter medications. Check with a qualified professional— your herbalist, physician, and/or pharmacist—about possible problems.

▼ If a minor condition does not respond to herbal treatment in two or three weeks, it is time to seek professional attention.

▼ Consult your physician and a qualified herbalist before you begin herbal treatment of any serious illness. Do not attempt self-diagnosis. Herbal treatment can effectively complement conventional medical treatment, but careful monitoring of your condition—as well as attention to possible interactions between drugs and herbal remedies—is necessary at all times.

▼ If you experience an allergic reaction to an herb, such as nausea or diarrhea, stop taking the remedy and immediately contact a qualified professional herbalist or your own physician.

▼ Many people use diuretics—including natural herbal ones—to lose weight. But diuretics are not the appropriate route to losing weight. A diet that is low in fat and calories and high in fiber, in conjunction with regular aerobic exercise, is the healthy and long-term formula for weight loss.

How to Find a Qualified Herbalist

Knowledgeable people at local health food stores and herb shops may be able to recommend a qualified herbalist. It's especially helpful to rely on the references of friends who have found an herbalist they like and trust. You can also visit holistic health centers, where herbalists are often available. Some people may feel most comfortable with an herbally oriented M.D.

Many herbalists have N.D. (Doctor of Naturopathy) degrees from a licensed school of naturopathy in the United States or Europe. The School of Medical Herbalism and its United States affiliates are among the most renowned trainers of herbalists. Feel free to talk to your herbalist about his or her qualifications and experience. Ask the herbalist for the names and numbers of patients he or she has treated for similar conditions. And keep in mind that the best herbalists are often home-grown.

A helpful address to write for further information is the American Herb Association, Box 353, Rescue, California, 95672. They may be able to steer you toward qualified herbalists in your area. Another excellent source of herbal information and how to find an herbal practitioner is the American Botanical Council, which also publishes *Herbal-Gram:* P.O. Box 201660, Austin, TX 78720; telephone: (800) 748-2617. The American Association of Naturopathic Physicians may be able to refer you to an herbally oriented doctor in your area: Box 20386, Seattle, Washington, 98102; telephone: (206) 323-7610.

Where to Purchase Herbal Remedies

Commercially prepared herbal remedies are widely available in health food markets and herb stores. Many pharmacies and major supermarket chains are also beginning to carry them. So instead of going through the painstaking process of growing and grinding your own herbs, you can stroll over to the health store or herb shop and choose from a wide variety of herbal combinations.

Remember to tuck this book in your bag when you go; as we told you in Chapter One, manufacturers are not allowed to make any healing claims for herbs, as it is not to their advantage to go through the FDA approval process.

Your best bet is to be an informed consumer. Carefully read the information in this book about each herb—its primary function and other benefits, the types of preparations and dosages, and any precautions you should take while using it—before you purchase a particular herb.

It is equally important to pay careful attention to the manufacturer's recommendations: different manufacturers may vary the combinations and amounts of herbs used in their remedies. Study the information on each herbal preparation; make sure there is detailed information on appropriate dosages. In a good health food store or herb shop, there should also be someone available to answer any further questions you may have.

Mail Order Sources of Herbs

Herbal remedies have yet to reach all corners of the United States, so you may find yourself stumped when it comes to acquiring the remedy you want. To fill this gap, many manufacturers now offer their herbal products by mail. Others only sell in bulk to wholesalers, but are happy to send you material about their products and information about where you can buy them in or near your area.

Some herbal manufacturers have free (800) numbers you can call; helpful and knowledgeable people are generally available to answer your questions and steer you in the right herbal direction. Write or call these manufacturers for a catalog, which is often free. Here are a few of the many companies that offer informational material, dried herbs, and/or herbal preparations by mail:

▼ Companion Plants
7247 North Coolville Ridge Road
Athens, OH 45701

▼ East-West Herb Products
65 Mechanic Street, Suite 103
Red Bank, NJ 07701

▼ Green Terrestrial
P.O. Box 41, Rte. 9W
Milton, NY 12547

▼ Health Center for Better Living
6189 Taylor Road
Naples, FL 33942
(Request "Useful Guide to Herbal Health
Care")

▼ The Herb and Spice Collection
P.O. Box 118
Norway, IA 52318
(800) 365-4372

▼ HerbPharm's Whole Herb Catalog
P.O. Box 116
Williams, OR 97544
(503) 846-6262

▼ Nature's Herbs
1010 Forty-sixth Street
Emeryville, CA 94608
(510) 601-0700

▼ Phyto-Pharmica
P.O. Box 1348
Green Bay, WI 54305

▼ Planetary Formulas
P.O. Box 533W
Soquel, CA 95073
(800) 776-7701

▼ Rainbow Light
207 McPherson Street
Department P
Santa Cruz, CA 95060
(800) 635-1233

▼ Rosemary House
120 South Market Street
Mechanicsburg, PA 17055

▼ Sage Mountain Herbal Products
P.O. Box 420
East Barre, VT 05649

▼ Taylor's Herb Gardens, Inc.
1535 Lone Oak Road
Vista, CA 92084

CHAPTER 3
Herbs for Optimum Health and Vitality

Legend has it that on his deathbed, the famous scientist Louis Pasteur, often considered the father of germ theory, pronounced that the germ is nothing—but the terrain is everything.

Just what did Pasteur mean by this statement? He meant that germs cannot invade healthy matter. Germs require an unhealthy environment. Germs thrive in decaying matter.

The herbal approach to good health is to head all those germs off at the pass. If our bodies are strong and vigorous, germs cannot gain a foothold. At the same time, many of the diseases that afflict us as we age are less likely to develop.

If you want to feel and look your best every day, try the herbal approach. In this chapter you'll find both general tips on healthy living and our favorite herbal tonics to nourish and support the many organs and systems that make up your body. A healthy lifestyle, including herbal support, is the surest route to a long and vital life.

The Changing Face of Disease

One hundred years ago, the average worldwide life expectancy was only about thirty-five years. Today we can easily expect to live to a ripe old age, surviving well into our seventies, eighties, nineties—a lucky few of us even

25

break the century mark! And yet more and more of us are beginning to worry: what quality of life will we enjoy as we add these decades to our lives? The answer to that question lies in our own hands: leading a healthy lifestyle today is the single most important thing we can all do to prevent disease and maintain good health and vitality as we age.

Drugs, environmental pollutants, pesticides, and inadequately tested food additives are all around us today. In addition to this attack from without, our bodies have been internally weakened through stress, and our resistance naturally dwindles as we age. Our immune systems have been bombarded with huge amounts of drugs—many via conventional medical channels, and others through the insidious infiltration of our food and water. Meat, poultry, eggs, and milk may all contain residues of chemicals and antibiotics. The consequence? Our immune systems no longer protect us as efficiently as they did in the past.

We need to start nurturing and caring for our bodies—and we need to start today. Every day new research confirms what nutritionists and epidemiologists have long suspected: the slow diseases that evolve in our bodies as we age—killers such as heart disease and many forms of cancer—can, like germs, be headed off at the pass. And the sooner we embrace a healthy lifestyle, the greater likelihood we will have of avoiding these diseases and living a long and healthy life.

The truth is that the more scientists learn about the active ingredients in herbs, fruits, vegetables, and beans, the more convinced they are that the powerful compounds in these plant foods can slow the bodily breakdown that leads inexorably to cancer and other chronic diseases. In addition to the well-known benefits of vitamins and fiber, plants are replete with chemicals that may block the initiation and growth of a wide variety of chronic diseases.

As our life-spans grow longer, the value of herbs rises far beyond that of simple cures for simple ailments. Herbs have significant long-term nourishing and sustaining effects on our bodies. Herbs can help you live a long life . . . and a full life.

What Are Herbal Tonics?

Herbal tonics are preparations that promote health and prevent disease. We take herbal tonics to support, nourish, and restore health and vitality to the different systems and organs of our bodies. In herbalism this effect is known as tonifying. When our bodies are in tone, we don't offer hospitality to any stray germs. We wake up in the morning ready to conquer the world.

There are different herbal combinations to keep each of the organs and systems in our bodies in tip-top form. Some herbs are especially supportive to our hearts; others boost our immune systems. A number of herbs are natural antioxidants, which means that they obliterate the free-radical molecules that can damage our cells and may eventually lead to both cancer and heart disease.

Many people have a weakness or susceptibility somewhere in their bodies, whether due to an unfortunate lifestyle choice (for example, smoking cigarettes or eating too many fatty foods) or because of a genetic predisposition (what we used to call a family history of a disease). Herbs can rally your body's defenses to help ward off your susceptibility to that disease—*before* you actually become ill with it.

Hawthorn berries are the classic heart restorative; if

your family has a history of high blood pressure or heart disease, you may want to consider a heart tonic that contains hawthorn berries. If you're one of the many women who suffer from chronic urinary-tract infections, drinking plenty of natural sugar-free cranberry juice might spare you a lot of discomfort—as well as costly medical bills. If you are plagued by cramps and muscle spasms, latch on to the very aptly named cramp bark.

Let's look at some tips for general good health, and explore some general herbal tonics that nurture and support the various systems and organs of our bodies. If you visit an herbalist, he or she may adjust these tonics to fit you as an individual.

Get Heart-Smart

Helpful herbs:

▼ Hawthorn berries
▼ Motherwort
▼ Dandelion leaves

A sound heart and circulatory system are the basis of good health. It's important to strengthen and tone your heart and the blood vessels that carry blood from your heart to all the vital organs of your body.

There are lifestyle choices you can make to naturally prevent problems from developing in your heart and circulatory system: regular aerobic exercise; a diet low in cholesterol, fat, and sodium; stress reduction; and avoiding habits such as smoking or drinking too much alcohol. These are simple steps we can all take to keep our hearts healthy.

There are also wonderful herbal tonics for your heart.

Heart tonics are especially good because they can be taken over long periods of time. Helpful herbs include hawthorn berries, which strengthen your heart muscle, and motherwort, which stabilizes the heart. Dandelion is a dandy diuretic useful for all types of circulation problems; diuretics improve circulation by reducing water buildup. Keep in mind, of course, that serious heart problems require medical attention.

An herbal tonic we recommend for your heart can be made from equal parts of hawthorn and motherwort. Put 1 teaspoon of the dried herbal combination or 3 teaspoons of the fresh herbs into 1 cup of boiling water. Cover and steep for 10 minutes. Drink up to 3 cups daily for three-month periods.

▲

The Way to a Healthy Heart
▼ Don't smoke.
▼ Maintain a desirable weight.
▼ Engage in regular aerobic exercise.
▼ Keep your blood pressure under control.
▼ Monitor your cholesterol level, which should remain below 200 mg/dl.
▼ Moderate your consumption of saturated fat, which is found in all animal products, including meat, poultry, eggs, and dairy. Saturated fat raises your blood cholesterol level more than anything else you eat.
▼ Increase your consumption of the ''good'' fat— omega-3 fatty acids, which are found in deep-sea

fish such as salmon and swordfish. Omega-3 is thought to lower blood cholesterol levels.
▼ Consume more dietary fiber and antioxidant nutrients from whole grains, fruits, and vegetables.

Boost Your Immune System

Helpful herbs:

▼ Astragalus
▼ Echinacea
▼ Red clover

In recent years our immune systems have become the target not only of AIDS but of an entire host of autoimmune diseases. While we don't know all the reasons for this change, it's probably because we live longer and under a greater degree of stress than in the past. In addition, our systems have been battered with a variety of antibiotics and other drugs, a process that eventually weakens our own natural defensive resources.

A diet rich in immune-boosting nutrients, regular exercise, the avoidance of negative habits, the maintenance of emotional health, and a general sense of well-being are all important ways of supporting your immune system. In fact, as you will see again and again, this simple recipe is really the key to good health for all your body's systems and organs.

There are many lovely herbal tonics that specifically support the body's immune system. One of our favorite immune boosters is the Chinese herb astragalus. Commercial preparations of astragalus are readily available in health food stores and herb shops; carefully follow the instructions on the label. We also recommend echinacea and red clover as valuable immune-enhancing herbs. You can make a tonic of them with equal parts of yellow dock and dandelion root, which help your body eliminate toxins. Boil the dandelion, echinacea, and yellow dock roots for 10 minutes. Add the flower heads of red clover, cover, and steep for another 10 minutes. Drink up to 3 cups daily. If you instead opt for the tincture, take up to 3 teaspoons daily.

Supporting Your Immune System

▼ Eat sensibly, including plenty of fruits, vegetables, legumes, and whole grains. This type of diet should be high in the following immune-strengthening nutrients: beta-carotene, vitamin E, vitamin C, vitamin B_6, folic acid, zinc, and selenium.

▼ Get in the habit of exercising regularly.

▼ Avoid habits that can compromise your immune system, such as cigarette smoking, excessive alcoholic intake, drug use, and multiple sexual partners without appropriate protection.

▼ Keep your chin up: try to maintain emotional stability and a positive outlook.

Improve Your Digestion

Helpful herbs, stimulants:

- ▼ Cardamom seeds
- ▼ Dandelion root
- ▼ Fenugreek
- ▼ Gentian

Helpful herbs, relaxants:

- ▼ Chamomile
- ▼ Hops
- ▼ Lemon balm
- ▼ Slippery elm

Most digestive difficulties can be sidestepped simply by maintaining a healthy lifestyle. Both alcohol and tobacco irritate the walls of your intestine and should be avoided. Tea and coffee, even decaffeinated, increase stomach acid and can cause an upset stomach. Likewise, stress and anxiety can pose unnecessary burdens on your digestive system.

On the positive side, eat plenty of fresh fruits, vegetables, whole grains, and beans. The natural fiber in these foods dilutes carcinogenic compounds in your colon and speeds them along through your digestive system. Fiber also discourages the growth of unhealthy bacteria; it helps your body eliminate toxins by bolstering the growth of benign bacteria, which crowd out the more harmful strains.

There are two kinds of herbal tonics for your digestion: stimulants and relaxants. Some people suffer from sluggish or weak digestion, and can benefit from a digestive stimulant. Others—especially you type A personalities out there —tend to have an irritated digestive tract; herbal relaxants are soothing remedies in these cases. If you're in doubt about which camp you're in, consult a qualified herbalist to see what remedy is most appropriate for you.

An effective digestive stimulant includes an equal combination of cardamom seeds, dandelion root, fenugreek, and gentian. Boil the dandelion and gentian roots for 10 minutes. Toss in the cardamom and fenugreek seeds, cover, and steep for another 10 minutes. Drink up to 3 cups daily for three months at a time; then take a break and start again.

We also recommend herbs such as chamomile, hops, and lemon balm to soothe your digestive tissue and reduce overactivity in your system. Make a relaxing digestive tonic by putting 1 teaspoon of this dried herbal combination or 3 teaspoons of the fresh herbs into 1 cup of boiling water. Cover and steep for 10 minutes, and drink up to 3 cups each day. Slippery elm is best to use in tablet form, so that it will pass through the stomach and get into the intestines.

▲

How to Support Your Digestion
▼ Don't smoke.
▼ If you drink alcohol, do so in moderation.
▼ Don't eat when angry or under stress.
▼ Include plenty of fresh fruits, fresh vegetables, whole grains, and beans in your diet—the fiber in these foods is your best natural defense against constipation.
▼ Avoid large meals.

▼ Reduce or eliminate your consumption of coffee
and tea.

Get Rid of the Toxins in Your Body
Helpful Herbs:

▼ Dandelion root
▼ Milk thistle
▼ Yellow dock root

Waste products and toxins are eliminated from our
bodies by the liver and kidneys. The liver is both the largest
and one of the most important organs in your body. It de-
toxifies alcohol, fat, and the other potentially damaging
substances that enter your body. Herbalists today are particularly sensitive to the needs of the liver, since its job has
been considerably stepped up in the polluted environment
in which we live.

There are many excellent tonics that nurture and tone
the liver. We recommend this nutritious and supportive
herbal tonic: equal parts of dandelion root, milk thistle, and
yellow dock root. Boil the dandelion and yellow dock roots
for 10 minutes. Toss in the milk thistle seeds, cover, and
steep for another 10 minutes, and drink up to 3 cups daily.
Serious liver problems, of course, require professional
treatment.

Your kidneys and urinary system are also prone to a
variety of infections, especially when your body's defenses
are low. Frequent use of antibiotics, poor diet, and constipation are common causes of problems in this system. The

herbs most frequently used to nourish and support the urinary system are diuretics, which increase urine flow.

There are many herbal diuretics to use when you retain water and are therefore unable to eliminate toxins. Most diuretics should not be taken on a long-term basis because they deplete the amount of potassium in your body. But dandelion leaves are a valuable exception here: the naturally high potassium content of dandelion leaves counteracts this side effect. Follow the directions on commercial dandelion remedies, beginning usage with the lowest recommended dosage. If you continue to suffer from kidney problems, it's time to pay a visit to your doctor.

▲

Support Your Liver and Kidneys

▼ Drink at least 8 glasses of water daily.

▼ Avoid caffeine.

▼ Consume alcohol in moderation only.

▼ Eat a variety of whole foods.

▼ Make sure you practice good hygiene.

▼ Avoid frequent use of antibiotics.

▼ Take time out from your busy life to rest. Try to eliminate excess stress from your life.

▼ Take vitamin C and eat yogurt to renew the beneficial bacteria that combat infections.

▼ Get plenty of exercise.

▼ Do not engage in risky behavior, such as unsafe sex or drug abuse (especially needle sharing, which is a major cause of hepatitis).

Breathe Easy

Helpful herbs, stimulants:

- ▼ Balm of Gilead
- ▼ Elecampane
- ▼ Lobelia

Helpful herbs, relaxants:

- ▼ Angelica
- ▼ Aniseed
- ▼ Coltsfoot
- ▼ Licorice
- ▼ Mullein

We each breathe enough air every day to blow up thousands of balloons. Every time we breathe, we inhale much-needed oxygen and exhale waste matter, carbon dioxide. A diet of whole foods, exercise, and fresh air are all keys to respiratory health. Although many of us live in urban areas where we are forced to breathe polluted air, we have the ability to avoid the greatest contaminant to our lungs: tobacco. Remember that you also have the right to say no to passive smoke. When others smoke around you they are unfairly jeopardizing *your* lungs.

There are two types of herbal remedies for the respiratory system, but many of the herbs—such as elecampane, licorice, and mullein—are reactively neutral and can be used in either category. If your lungs are clogged with mucus and phlegm, we recommend stimulating expectorants such as balm of Gilead and elecampane. When the lungs have been taxed with over-activity and tension, respiratory relaxants—including aniseed, coltsfoot, and mullein—are appropriate.

Lobelia is a valuable all-around lung tonic. A helpful herbal combination consists of 1 part elecampane, 1 part lobelia, and 2 parts licorice. Boil the elecampane and licorice roots for 10 minutes. Add the aboveground parts of lobelia, cover, and steep for another 10 minutes. Drink up to 3 cups daily.

▲

How to Strengthen Your Lungs

▼ Don't smoke. And don't tolerate breathing the passive smoke of others. Studies increasingly show that passive smoke can also be bad for your health.

▼ Eat a well-balanced, vitamin-packed diet.

▼ Support your lung power by getting lots of aerobic exercise.

▼ Get plenty of fresh air. While we all can't live in the country, caution should be exercised in the cities that have pollution problems. Small children and the elderly, for example, are advised to take it easy or stay inside on those stifling smog-alert days that many cities experience each summer.

▼ Use a humidifier in winter.

▼ If you have respiratory allergies, avoid exposure to pollen, mold spores, house dust, and other common triggers.

Nourish Your Reproductive System and Add Sexual Vigor

Helpful herbs for women:

▼ Agnus-castus (*vitex*)
▼ False unicorn root
▼ Black haw

Helpful herbs for men:

▼ Damiana
▼ Ginseng
▼ Saw palmetto

Healthy children are born to women and men who lead healthy lives. While traditionally the emphasis has been on the woman's lifestyle, increasing evidence shows that a father's lifestyle also has an impact on the health of his newborn child. A well-balanced diet, regular exercise, and a stress-free, loving, and nurturing emotional environment lead to healthy and successful pregnancies.

There are many herbs that strengthen and tone women's reproductive systems. They include agnus-castus, black haw, and false unicorn root. Damiana, ginseng, and saw palmetto act as tonics for men's reproductive systems. One note of caution: If you are or suspect you may be pregnant, talk to a qualified herbalist and/or your physician before using herbal remedies.

There are also a number of herbal combinations that are taken to increase fertility. These should be used at the rate of 3 cups a day for a period of three months. If you are still experiencing problems after this period, you may want to consult a qualified professional. It's possible that there is a physical problem that needs to be corrected, especially if you have been unsuccessfully trying to conceive for a long time.

An herbal combination we recommend to enhance women's fertility consists of dong quai, false unicorn, and raspberry leaf. Boil the dong quai and false unicorn roots for 10 minutes. Add the aboveground portion of raspberry leaf, cover, and steep for an additional 10 minutes.

There are a number of herbs that stimulate the uterus and should be avoided if you are trying to become pregnant. These include barberry, goldenseal, juniper, pennyroyal, and sage. When in doubt, contact a qualified professional.

Asian or Siberian ginseng, damiana, and saw palmetto are the fertility herbs that we recommend to male clients. Boil the ginseng root for 10 minutes. Add the aboveground parts of damiana and saw palmetto, cover, and steep for another 10 minutes.

Traditional societies have also long touted the ability of various herbs to add sexual vigor. But the truth of the matter, according to most modern herbalists, is that there are no magic love potions out there. The desire and ability to enjoy sex is linked instead with your overall sense of well-being. When your body is healthy and your mind is at peace, you simply don't have to worry about it. In the meantime, if you'd like to try out some of the herbs that have traditionally been thought of as aphrodisiacs, astragalus, burdock, damiana, dong quai, false unicorn, ginseng, and kava are all reputed sexual stimulants.

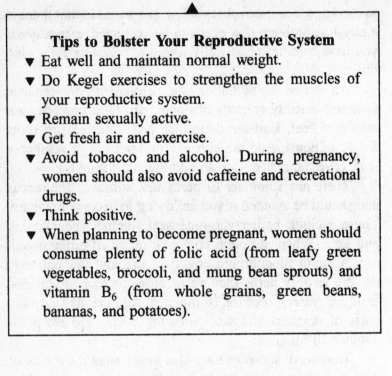

Tips to Bolster Your Reproductive System

▼ Eat well and maintain normal weight.

▼ Do Kegel exercises to strengthen the muscles of your reproductive system.

▼ Remain sexually active.

▼ Get fresh air and exercise.

▼ Avoid tobacco and alcohol. During pregnancy, women should also avoid caffeine and recreational drugs.

▼ Think positive.

▼ When planning to become pregnant, women should consume plenty of folic acid (from leafy green vegetables, broccoli, and mung bean sprouts) and vitamin B_6 (from whole grains, green beans, bananas, and potatoes).

Get on Top of Stress

Your nervous system is an important part of the physical makeup of your body. In order to be wholly healthy, we must pay close attention to our emotional health as well as to elements such as nutrition and exercise. Too many of us lead lives filled with stress and anxiety, and this stress has a negative impact on our overall health.

We must take steps to reduce the levels of stress in our lives, and we can do this by making changes in our lifestyle. Exercise, for example, is one of the best stress reducers. It's also important not to suppress your anger; try to talk out your difficulties. You must identify the source of your stress. Is it a relationship? Your job? Either reduce the stress from that source, or eliminate the source from your life.

Mild herbal remedies can also help you relax. Valerian, hops, and damiana all help relieve tension. But the truth is that neither exercise nor herbs will do the trick alone—the bottom line is that you must deal with the issues in your life that are creating or underlying your stress.

A soothing herbal tonic may contain equal parts of damiana, hops, and valerian. Boil the valerian root for 10 minutes. Add the aboveground parts of damiana and hops, cover, and steep for an additional 10 minutes. Since this remedy makes some people sleepy, avoid driving or operating heavy machinery while using it. While you may drink up to 3 cups a day, begin with one cup after dinner and gradually increase your dosage as needed.

Stress-Busters

We believe that you should accept your emotions —without getting stuck on them. If you have to, close the windows of your car and scream! Just get stress out of your system in whatever way works best for you.

- ▼ Exercise.
- ▼ Meditation.
- ▼ Yoga.
- ▼ Deep breathing.
- ▼ Biofeedback.
- ▼ Take a hot bath.

▼ Read a good book.
▼ Go out to the movies.
▼ Listen to your favorite music.
▼ Talk to a friend.
▼ Get a pet.

Look Your Best

Healthy skin comes from the inside out. Your skin is actually a very good indicator of your general health. A healthy lifestyle is your first step to healthy skin. Your skin —as well as the rest of you—will benefit from a nutritious diet, fresh air, exercise, sleep, and relaxation.

Many women also choose herbal cosmetics as a safe, natural, and inexpensive alternative to commercial cosmetics, which often contain chemicals that can harm your skin. Several of the ingredients from which you can make your own cosmetics are probably already on your kitchen shelf.

Mix an infusion of fennel with plain yogurt, and you have a natural skin cleanser. Or try an herbal skin tonic to revive dull and tired skin: make an infusion of chamomile and lavender flowers, and rub it on your face and body. Other quick facial pick-me-ups include dandelion, horsetail, nettle, rosemary, sage, and thyme. Or give yourself a facial steambath—put 10 drops of peppermint oil in 2 quarts of hot water, cover your head with a towel, and lean over the pot.

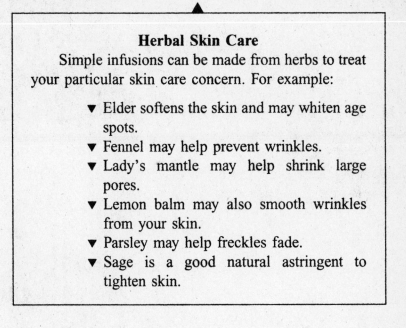

Herbal Skin Care

Simple infusions can be made from herbs to treat your particular skin care concern. For example:

- ▼ Elder softens the skin and may whiten age spots.
- ▼ Fennel may help prevent wrinkles.
- ▼ Lady's mantle may help shrink large pores.
- ▼ Lemon balm may also smooth wrinkles from your skin.
- ▼ Parsley may help freckles fade.
- ▼ Sage is a good natural astringent to tighten skin.

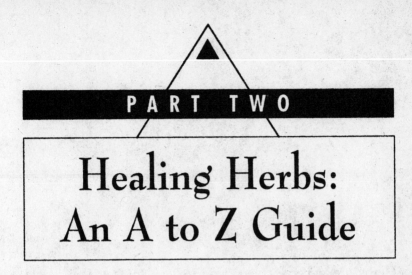

PART TWO

Healing Herbs: An A to Z Guide

Herbs are generally very safe to use. In fact, you would have to take an enormous dose of most herbs before experiencing any side effects. Nonetheless, caution should be exercised when using any remedy; refer to page 18 for safety guidelines when using herbs. If any additional safety information is required before taking any of the herbs we have included here, you will find it in the precaution section of that particular herb.

▲

AGNUS-CASTUS (*Vitex agnus-castus*)

Agnus-castus, also known as vitex, chasteberry, chaste tree, or monk's pepper, is a restorative herb used to treat menopause and PMS. It is an effective, all-around balancing herb for women. For centuries this has been a popular herb in Europe, and today agnus-castus is a growing favorite in the United States.

Agnus-castus is a safe and natural alternative to hormone-replacement therapy, which many middle-aged women currently choose to counter the effects of menopause. Agnus-castus, or vitex, is one of our favorite herbs. We use it in almost all our menopausal remedies.

Parts Used: Fruit.

Primary Functions

▼ Agnus-castus alleviates many menstrual problems, including PMS.

▼ Agnus-castus counters many of the unpleasant symptoms of menopause, including hot flashes, night sweats, and anxiety.

Other Benefits

▼ Agnus-castus naturally stimulates the production of progesterone.

▼ Agnus-castus may be effective in reducing fibroid tumors.

▼ Agnus-castus may increase milk production in nursing mothers. (Check first with a qualified professional.)

Preparation and Dosage

Agnus-castus products are most commonly available in commercial form as capsules, extracts, and tinctures.

Capsules: 1 capsule up to three times daily.

Extract: Mix 10 to 30 drops in water or juice up to three times daily.

Tincture: 1 teaspoon up to three times daily.

General Precautions

Agnus-castus is a very safe herb. As with all gynecological herbs, women who wish to use agnus-castus should first consult with a qualified professional if they are or suspect they may be pregnant. Since agnus castus is a hormonal remedy, it is inappropriate for use in children.

▲

AGRIMONY (*Agrimonia eupatoria*)

Agrimony, also known as sticklewort or cocklebur, is an astringent herb; that is, it has binding qualities that can stop bleeding. Agrimony is also used to treat urinary infections and infections of the intestinal tract. It is a restorative tonic to the stomach. Some researchers have also noted that agrimony has antiviral properties. Ointments made from agrimony may shrink your hemorrhoids and soothe sores and insect bites.

Parts Used: Aboveground parts.

Primary Functions

▼ Agrimony has strong astringent qualities, which make this herb especially useful in many cases of bleeding.

▼ Agrimony may be especially helpful in treating vaginal bleeding (often associated with menopause) and vaginal discharges. (Some commercial preparations to stop bleeding combine agrimony with cinnamon bark and yarrow.)

Other Benefits

▼ Agrimony can restore tone to the intestines and stomach.

▼ Externally, ointments made from agrimony may be used to treat hemorrhoids, athlete's foot, insect bites, and sores.

Preparation and Dosage

Agrimony products are most commonly available as capsules, decoctions, tinctures, and ointments.

Capsules: 5 to 10 #0 capsules up to three times daily.

Decoction: 3 to 5 tablespoons up to four times daily.

Tincture: 1 teaspoon up to three times daily.

Ointment: Apply as needed.

General Precautions

Agrimony is a very safe herb. Yet in the treatment of vaginal discharges, women should consult with their physician if the discharge is full of pus or green.

ALFALFA (*Medicago sativa*)

Alfalfa, also known as lucerne, is a nutritious and restorative tonic. In addition to the alkaloids asparagine and trigonelline, alfalfa is rich in beta-carotene, vitamins C, D, E, and K, and minerals such as calcium, potassium, magnesium, and iron.

The Arabs, who discovered alfalfa, named it "the father of all foods." Alfalfa is an excellent overall tonic; it can be used to boost your normal vitality and strength, and it is especially helpful during convalescence or anemia. Exciting new research suggests that alfalfa may reduce blood cholesterol levels and plaque deposits, which precede heart disease and stroke. Another study suggests that alfalfa may neutralize carcinogens in the colon.

Parts Used: Leaves.

Primary Functions

▼ Alfalfa is an excellent source of beta-carotene and other valuable vitamins and nutrients.

▼ Alfalfa can stimulate your appetite and help you gain weight. This can be a boon to those convalescing from a disease, suffering from an immune disorder, or simply going through the ordinary process of aging.

Other Benefits

▼ Alfalfa may be used to treat acute or chronic cystitis.

▼ Alfalfa can relieve inflammation of the prostate.

▼ Alfalfa may ease lower-back pain and reduce bloating or water retention.

▼ Alfalfa can relieve constipation.

▼ Alfalfa may alleviate the symptoms of rheumatism and arthritis.

▼ If you are a nursing mother, alfalfa may increase the flow of your breast milk. (Check first with a qualified professional.)

Preparation and Dosage

Alfalfa products are most commonly available in commercial form as capsules and teas. Although alfalfa leaves are more significant than sprouts in herbal healing, you can't go wrong by simply tossing some fresh alfalfa sprouts on your salad.

Capsules: 3 to 6 capsules daily.

Teas: May be taken up to three times daily.

General Precautions

No one should eat alfalfa seeds, which contain a toxic amino acid. Enjoy the sprouts in moderation—but don't overdo. Otherwise, alfalfa is a very safe herb, and only normal precautions need be taken. If the dosage on the label is stated in terms of a range, begin use with the lowest dosage.

▲

ALMOND (*Prunus amygdalus*)

The kernel from the almond plant provides us with a safe and natural alternative to dry commercial soaps and shampoos. Oil made from almonds has natural skin-nourishing qualities. Recent studies have also suggested that almond oil—like olive oil—when incorporated into your diet may help lower your total cholesterol level.

Parts Used: Kernel and oil.

Primary Functions

▼ Almond soaps can clean your skin without making it dry.

▼ Almond oils and lotions will soften and moisturize your skin.

Other Benefits

▼ Cooking with almond oil may reduce your cholesterol level.

Preparation and Dosage

Almond products are most commonly available in commercial form as nut kernels, oils, lotions, and butters.

Kernels: You can make your own mask at home for dry skin by finely grinding almonds and adding a little milk to make a paste. Pat the mixture gently on your face (don't try to rub it in) and leave on for half an hour.

Oil, Lotion, and Butter: Apply liberally as needed.

General Precautions

The external use of almond products is very safe. However, if you are prone to allergies, you may want to try an almond product on a small patch of your skin before widely applying it. The same is true for using almond oil in your cooking. If you think you may be allergic to it, start with a very small amount. If you experience no allergic reactions, feel free to use almond products on a regular basis.

▲

ALOE VERA (*Aloe barbadenis*)

Although there are over two hundred varieties of this remarkable herb, aloe vera (or "true aloe" in Latin) is widely considered the most effective type of aloe. This versatile herb has been used for more than thirty-five hundred years.

Taken internally, aloe vera can relieve constipation and benefit the liver. Externally, the gel taken from the leaf of the aloe plant is one of nature's greatest moisturizers.

In Ayurvedic medicine aloe vera gel is known as estrogenic, or having significant tonic and restorative qualities for women. In Sanskrit the gel is called *kumari;* the translation is "goddess," again referring to its tonic, antiaging value for women.

Aloe can also be used to relieve sunburn and promote the healing of other kinds of minor burns and skin irritations. Recent studies in the United States have indicated that it may be useful in relieving radiation burns suffered by patients undergoing chemotherapy.

Parts Used: Juice from the leaves.

Primary Functions
▼ Taken internally, aloe vera is a laxative and a restorative to the liver.

▼ Applied externally, aloe vera can relieve the pain and promote the healing of minor burns, wounds, and skin irritations.

Other Benefits

▼ Aloe vera is a natural moisturizer.

▼ Aloe vera has been used to treat radiation burns.

▼ Aloe vera may help slow the development of wrinkles.

Preparation and Dosage

Aloe vera products are most commonly available in commercial form as capsules and gels.

Capsules: 1 capsule up to three times daily.

Gel: Apply liberally as needed.

Special Precautions

Aloe should never be taken internally during pregnancy, as it may lead to miscarriage. Aloe should not be taken internally by children.

The external application of aloe vera is safe and natural. However, some commercial aloe products may include perfumes or other ingredients to which you may be allergic; always read the label before purchasing an aloe vera preparation.

ANGELICA (*Angelica archangelica*)

Angelica is a versatile herb useful as a general tonic for good health as well as a remedy for a variety of ailments. It is said to be named after the Archangel Raphael, who gave this herb to a monk during the plague epidemic. Candied stems of angelica are often eaten in Europe, especially around the holidays.

Angelica promotes circulation and warms the body. It is used to relieve stomachaches, indigestion, and menstrual cramps in women. Angelica is often a part of the herbal treatment of colds, coughs, flus, and fevers. Applied externally, angelica can ease rheumatic pains, stomach cramps, and muscle spasms.

Parts Used: Leaves and roots.

Primary Functions

▼ Angelica is a good all-around tonic.

▼ Angelica improves circulation.

▼ Angelica can be used by anemics to promote circulation to otherwise chilly hands and feet.

Other Benefits

▼ Angelica can help regulate the menstrual cycle.

▼ Angelica has a warming influence on the body.

▼ Angelica can reduce lung congestion, as in colds, coughs, flus, and fevers.

▼ Angelica is a good expectorant.

▼ Angelica can relieve stomach cramps, indigestion, gas, and heartburn.

▼ Angelica can ease rheumatic pains.

Preparation and Dosage

Angelica products are most commonly available in commercial form as capsules, tinctures, and liniments.

Capsules: 1 capsule up to three times daily.

Tincture: 1 teaspoon up to three times daily.

Liniment: Apply liberally as needed.

Special Precautions

Angelica should *never* be taken internally during pregnancy, as it may cause miscarriage. Diabetics should not use angelica, since it may increase blood sugar and cause weakness.

The external application of angelica is safe and natural. However, some commercial angelica products may include perfumes or other ingredients to which you may be allergic; always read the label before purchasing an angelica preparation.

ANISEED (*Pimpinella anisum*)

Aniseed has been used since ancient Egyptian times for its licorice flavor and as a remedy for digestive disorders, colds, and colic. It was one of the world's first perfumes. The volatile oil in aniseed is what makes it especially effective in treating colic and flatulence. Externally applied, aniseed may be useful in getting rid of scabies and lice.

Parts Used: Dried seeds.

Primary Functions

▼ Aniseed is an excellent remedy for flatulence (gas) and colic.

▼ Aniseed can aid digestion.

▼ Aniseed may relieve nausea, bloating, belching, and stomach cramps.

Other Benefits

▼ Aniseed is used in the treatment of coughs, colds, whooping cough, and bronchial infections.

▼ Aniseed has a warming influence on the body.

▼ If you are a nursing mother, aniseed may increase the flow of your breast milk.

▼ Aniseed oil may be applied locally to treat lice or scabies infestations.

▼ Chewing a few seeds may relieve bad breath.

Preparation and Dosage

Aniseed products are most commonly available in commercial form as seeds, teas, and oils.

Seeds: Chew up to ½ ounce of the seeds each day. You can toast or roast the seeds and they're very tasty.

Tea: May be taken up to three times daily.

Oil: Apply locally as needed.

General Precautions

Aniseed is a very safe herb, but normal precautions should be taken with any remedy.

ARNICA (*Arnica montana*)

Arnica, also known as leopard's bane or wolf's bane, is available as an oil or liniment for the treatment of bruises, aches, strains, and swellings. In fact, many commercially prepared liniments contain arnica. This herb is appropriate for use on injuries only when the skin has not been broken, and you should discontinue its use at the first sign of any rash development. Arnica should *never* be taken internally—it may be toxic.

Parts Used: Flower heads.

Primary Functions

▼ Arnica can help heal painful bruises, aches, strains, and swellings.

▼ Arnica may be useful in the treatment of the joint inflammation associated with arthritis, rheumatism, and phlebitis.

Preparation and Dosage

Arnica products are most commonly available in commercial form as oils and liniments.

Oil or Liniment: Apply externally as needed. Withdraw treatment at the first sign of a rash.

Special Precautions

Arnica is a very helpful herb, but special precautions must be taken with its use. Arnica is not appropriate for internal use. It is toxic if taken internally, and overdoses can be fatal.

While arnica is a good healing agent for bruises, it should never be used externally on injuries in which the skin has been broken. If you experience a rash as a reaction to the application of arnica, discontinue its use immediately.

The homeopathic usage of arnica is very different from its herbal usage; in a homeopathic remedy, it is a much more refined substance and does not contain the toxic elements otherwise found.

▲

ARTICHOKE (*Cynara scolymus*)

Artichokes can be eaten freshly steamed or you can use the dried leaves, stem, or root for a healthy treat. Artichokes stimulate the flow of bile from the liver and are used in the treatment of liver disease. They have also been utilized in some forms of kidney disease, diabetes mellitus, and atherosclerosis. Eating artichokes can reduce your cholesterol level. The artichoke is also a natural diuretic, which means eating artichokes can help you reduce excess water weight. Artichokes even enjoy a reputation (scientifically unproven) for being an aphrodisiac.

Parts Used: Stem, leaves, and root.

Primary Functions
▼ Artichoke enhances liver function and is used in the treatment of chronic liver disease.

Other Benefits

▼ Artichoke reduces your cholesterol level (if you don't drench it in butter).

▼ Artichoke alleviates excess water weight.

▼ Artichoke may be effective in the treatment of certain kidney diseases, diabetes mellitus, and atherosclerosis.

Preparation and Dosage

Artichoke products are most commonly available in commercial form fresh or dried.

Fresh: Cut the stem and trim the tough outer leaves of the artichoke. Steam for 30 to 40 minutes, and serve with olive oil or lemon juice.

Dried: Prepare a tea with 1 to 4 grams of the dried leaves, stem, or root; take up to three times daily.

General Precautions

The use of fresh artichokes is safe and natural, but normal precautions should be taken with any remedy.

▲

ASPARAGUS ROOT (*Asparagus officinalis*)

While young asparagus shoots are a favorite springtime food, it is the asparagus root that has long been treasured by herbalists of China and India. Today it is increasingly popular in the Western world as well.

In traditional Chinese medicine, the asparagus root is known as a yin tonic; small doses taken regularly are believed to enhance feelings of love and compassion. In India, where the asparagus root is called *shatavari,* it is taken by women as a hormonal tonic. Asparagus root contains steroidal glycosides, which may account for its reputation for increasing positive feelings such as love, patience, and compassion.

In Western medicine asparagus root is used for its diuretic qualities; that is, it increases the flow of urine. It is a urinary-tract soother and tonic. In addition, asparagus root is a nutritive tonic that relieves some of the symptoms of chronic fatigue syndrome, tuberculosis, and even AIDS.

Parts Used: Root.

Primary Functions

▼ Asparagus root is a restorative tonic for the female reproductive system.

▼ Asparagus root may enhance fertility, relieve menstrual cramps, and increase the flow of breast milk in nursing women.

▼ Asparagus root is an effective treatment for urinary-tract infections and kidney stones.

Other Benefits

▼ Asparagus root may relieve painful swelling associated with rheumatism.

▼ The diuretic characteristics of asparagus root can help ease bloating and excess water weight.

▼ Asparagus root is a nutritive tonic for the lungs, making this herb useful in alleviating some of the wasting symptoms of tuberculosis and AIDS.

▼ Asparagus root may relieve throat dryness.

▼ Asparagus root is a good tonic for treating chronic fatigue syndrome and relieving general exhaustion.

Preparation and Dosage

Asparagus root products are most commonly available in commercial form as juices and decoctions.

Juice: 1 to 3 tablespoons of fresh juice up to three times daily.

Decoction: Boil 6 to 15 grams of asparagus root in water for 10 to 15 minutes, taken daily.

General Precautions

Asparagus root is a very safe herb, but normal precautions should be taken with any remedy.

▲

ASTRAGALUS (*Astragalus membranaceous*)

Astragalus is an ancient Chinese herb used to increase resistance to disease and to treat ailments such as diabetes, heart disease, and hypertension. It has a warming influence on your body and a tonic effect on many of the body organs. As with most Chinese herbs, astragalus is usually used in combination with other herbs.

Parts Used: Root.

Primary Functions

▼ Astragalus is a valuable tonic for increasing energy and resistance to disease.

▼ Astragalus may help activate the body's natural immune system.

Other Benefits

▼ Astragalus is a restorative tonic used in the treatment of various exhausting and wasting diseases.

▼ Astragalus is a diuretic that can help you rid your body of excess water weight.

▼ Under medical supervision, astragalus is sometimes given to patients undergoing chemotherapy.

Preparation and Dosage

Astragalus is most commonly available in commercial form as capsules, extracts, and tinctures.

Capsules: 1 400-milligram capsule up to three times daily.

Extract: Take as directed.

Tincture: Take 1 teaspoon up to three times daily.

General Precautions

Astragalus is a very safe herb, but normal precautions should be taken with any remedy.

BALM OF GILEAD (*Populus gileadensis*)

Balm of Gilead is an herb taken from tall poplar trees and used in the treatment of coughs and upper-respiratory infections. This herb indeed acts as a soothing balm to your body's mucous membranes. Balm of Gilead, which is often combined with the classic cough suppressant coltsfoot, is frequently mentioned in the Bible.

Parts Used: Closed buds.

Primary Functions

▼ Balm of Gilead can relieve laryngitis, coughs, and sore throats.

▼ Balm of Gilead is a soothing and disinfecting expectorant.

▼ Balm of Gilead is used in the treatment of bronchial and upper-respiratory infections.

Preparation and Dosage

Balm of Gilead is most commonly available in commercial form as a syrup or tincture. The correct dosage is the equivalent of 1 to 4 dried grams up to three times a day.

Syrup: 1 tablespoon up to three times daily.

Tincture: 1 teaspoon up to three times daily.

General Precautions

Balm of Gilead is a very safe herb, but normal precautions should be taken with any remedy.

BARBERRY (*Berberis vulgaris*)

Barberry, also known as jaundice berry, contains the infection-fighting constituent berberine. Its antibiotic qualities make barberry valuable in the treatment of ailments such as sore throats, diarrhea, and urinary-tract infections.

We recommend barberry for gall bladder infections and liver problems. In this way it acts as an effective and inexpensive substitute for goldenseal. Barberry is also a good tonic for digestion.

Parts Used: Bark of root or stem.

Primary Functions

▼ Barberry has valuable antibiotic qualities.

▼ Barberry may be one of the best liver and gall bladder remedies. It enhances the flow of bile through the liver, thus improving overall liver function.

Other Benefits

▼ Barberry may be useful in the treatment of sore throats, diarrhea, and urinary-tract and vaginal yeast infections.

▼ Barberry may help stimulate the immune system.

▼ Barberry may be helpful in relieving the symptoms of liver diseases such as hepatitis, jaundice, and chronic liver disease.

▼ Barberry may help detoxify the liver, as in cases of alcoholism, poor diet, or drug abuse.

▼ Barberry may also relieve spleen enlargement and some chronic stomach problems.

Preparation and Dosage

Barberry products are most commonly available in commercial form as capsules, decoctions, or tinctures.

Capsules: 2 to 5 #0 capsules up to three times daily.

Decoction: Up to 1 cup daily.

Tincture: ½ teaspoon to 1 teaspoon up to three times daily.

Special Precautions

Barberry should never be taken during pregnancy. Barberry is bitter and should be taken in small doses. Large doses may cause side effects such as nausea, vomiting, and a drop in blood pressure. For these reasons, barberry is best used under the supervision of a qualified herbalist or herbally oriented physician.

▲

BAYBERRY (*Myrica cerifera*)

Bayberry—also known as waxberry, candleberry, and wax myrtle—contains the antibiotic chemical myricitrin, which may fight a wide range of bacteria. Its antibiotic properties make bayberry useful in the treatment of diarrhea and in reducing fever. Bayberry may also be helpful for a variety of other ailments.

Parts Used: Bark of root.

Primary Functions

▼ Bayberry is used in the treatment of digestive

ailments, such as diarrhea, food poisoning, chronic gastritis, and dysentery. (It is often combined with ginger for the treatment of digestive problems.)

▼ Bayberry can help reduce fever.

Other Benefits

▼ Gargling with bayberry mouthwash will soothe sore throats and gums.

▼ The local application of bayberry is useful in healing wounds.

▼ A hot bayberry compress can be applied over varicose veins to strengthen blood vessels; it may also be helpful in treating hemorrhoids.

Preparation and Dosage

Bayberry is most commonly available in commercial form as capsules, extracts, and mouthwashs. A hot compress may be made by pouring hot bayberry tea on a towel. (Be careful that the tea is not so hot it burns you.)

Capsules: 1 capsule up to three times daily.

Extract: ½ teaspoon to 1 teaspoon as needed.

Mouthwash: As necessary.

Hot Compress: Apply to varicose veins or hemorrhoids as needed.

General Precautions

Bayberry is a very safe herb, but normal precautions should be taken with any remedy. Large doses of bayberry can cause nausea and vomiting, so it's best to avoid excessive use.

BISTORT (*Polygonum bistorta*)

Bistort—also known as adderwort, dragon weed, English serpentary, or snakeweed—is an astringent herb; that is, it has binding qualities that can stop bleeding. Bistort is a powerful digestive remedy, and it is also used as a mouthwash to combat gum disease and a douche to treat vaginal discharge.

Parts Used: Rhizome and root.

Primary Functions
▼ Bistort is a powerful astringent. It can help stop bleeding of all kinds.

▼ Bistort is an effective treatment for digestive disorders such as diarrhea, colitis, diverticulitis, and dysentery.

Other Benefits
▼ Use bistort mouthwash to treat gum disease.

▼ A bistort douche can counteract vaginal discharge.

Preparation and Dosage
Bistort is most commonly available in commercial form as capsules, teas, extracts, tinctures, douches, and mouthwashs.

Capsules: 1 to 5 #0 capsules up to three times daily.

Tea: May be taken several times daily.

Extract: ½ teaspoon to 1 teaspoon up to three times daily.

Tincture: 1 teaspoon up to three times daily.

Douche: When needed. (See "General Precautions" below.)

Mouthwash: As necessary.

General Precautions

In general, douches should not be used too regularly; if the condition you are treating with a douche persists, consult your doctor or herbalist. Never use a douche if you are pregnant.

▲

BLACK COHOSH (*Cimicifuga racemosa*)

Black cohosh—also known as black snakeroot, bugbane, and rattleroot—is a traditional Algonquian remedy for nervous conditions and women's health problems. It is a powerful antispasmodic herb; that is, it is an all-around muscle relaxer. Black cohosh is often used to relieve cramps, labor pains during childbirth, neuralgia, and generalized tension. Black cohosh improves circulation and is effective in the treatment of respiratory problems and rheumatism.

Parts Used: Dried rhizome and root.

Primary Functions

▼ Black cohosh has long been used by Native American women to bring on menstrual flow and relieve menstrual cramps.

▼ Black cohosh is used to treat a wide range of

nervous conditions, including insomnia, neuralgia (such as migraine headaches), numbness, and convulsions.

▼ Black cohosh relieves muscle spasms.

Other Benefits

▼ Black cohosh, when combined with blue cohosh, can help to bring on labor in pregnant women who are ready to deliver. (See "Special Precautions" below.)

▼ Black cohosh is often combined with herbs such as chamomile to ease menstrual and labor pains.

▼ Black cohosh is sometimes used to treat hypertension by helping to open blood vessels and equalize circulation.

▼ Black cohosh combined with herbs such as coltsfoot and yerba santa is effective in the treatment of asthma, bronchitis, and coughs.

▼ Black cohosh can help relieve the pain and swelling associated with rheumatism and arthritis.

Preparation and Dosage

Black cohosh is a very powerful herb; it is best taken under the supervision of a qualified herbalist or an herbally trained physician. Pay close attention to the "Special Precautions" below before using black cohosh; note especially the precautions about not using it during pregnancy. Black cohosh is most commonly available in commercial form as capsules, tinctures, and extracts.

Capsules: 1 capsule up to three times daily.

Tincture: 1 teaspoon up to 3 times daily.

Extract: Mix 10 to 30 drops of extract in water or juice, taken daily.

Special Precautions

This powerful herb is an excellent remedy but is best used under the supervision of a qualified natural herbalist or herbally oriented obstetrician or midwife.

Black cohosh brings on menstruation and labor; *never* take black cohosh during the course of your pregnancy, as it can cause miscarriage.

Your obstetrician or midwife, in consultation with a qualified herbalist, may use black cohosh to bring on and ease labor when your baby is full-term; but *never* attempt to make these determinations yourself. Black cohosh should only be used under close medical supervision. Black cohosh should be taken in small doses. An overdose can cause nausea and vomiting.

▲

BLACK HAW (*Viburnum prunifolium*)

Black haw, also known as sweet viburnum, is a traditional Native American remedy for women's gynecological problems. This herb contains the uterine relaxant scopoletin, and is widely used to soothe menstrual cramps. Closely related to cramp bark, black haw is often combined with cramp bark and false unicorn root in herbal remedies for women.

For centuries, black haw was taken to ward off threats of miscarriage. Today, however, there is some controversy about this practice, stemming from the fact that black haw also contains an aspirinlike chemical called salicin.

Parts Used: Dried bark of root, stem, or trunk.

Primary Functions
▼ Black haw is a tonic and sedative to the female reproductive system.

▼ Black haw is a powerful uterine relaxant. Its antispasmodic qualities make it an excellent treatment for menstrual cramps.

Other Benefits
▼ Because black haw contains the pain reliever salicin, it may be appropriate to use in the relief of headaches, arthritis, fever, and other pain.

▼ Black haw may be helpful in reducing high blood pressure, due to its relaxant and sedative actions.

▼ Black haw, an antispasmodic herb, may be effective in the treatment of asthma.

Preparation and Dosage
Black haw is most commonly available in commercial form as capsules, decoctions, and tinctures.

Capsules: 5 to 10 #0 capsules up to three times daily.

Decoction: Boil 2 teaspoons of dried bark in 1 cup of water for 10 minutes. Drink up to 3 cups a day. Try adding a little lemon or honey to offset the bitter taste of black haw.

Tincture: 1 teaspoon up to three times daily.

General Precautions
Many herbalists recommend black haw to pregnant clients to prevent miscarriage. But since it contains a small

amount of the aspirinlike pain reliever salicin, some pregnant women prefer not to use black haw.

▲

BLESSED THISTLE (*Cnicus benedictus*)

Blessed thistle is a traditional folk· remedy used in the treatment of stomach, liver, lung, and kidney problems. Because the liver is often affected by menstrual disorders, blessed thistle is also taken by women to correct the hormonal imbalances that lead to irregular menstrual cycles. Blessed thistle can improve your appetite, stimulate your memory, and act as an all-around tonic for your circulation and digestion.

Parts Used: Dried aboveground parts and seeds.

Primary Functions
▼ Blessed thistle can improve your digestion and relieve stomach cramps, indigestion, and gas.

▼ Blessed thistle can stimulate your appetite; thus it can help in treating anorexia.

Other Benefits
▼ Blessed thistle is used in the treatment of liver disorders such as jaundice and hepatitis.

▼ Blessed thistle may help lower fevers.

▼ Blessed thistle is used to stop bleeding and resolve blood clots.

▼ Women often take commercial preparations

containing blessed thistle and other gynecological herbs; these can correct the hormonal imbalances that may lead to irregular menstrual cycles and menstrual discomfort.

Preparation and Dosage

Blessed thistle products are most commonly available in commercial form as capsules and extracts. Many commercial preparations for women combine blessed thistle with other herbs, such as cramp bark and false unicorn root.

Capsules: 1 capsule up to three times daily.

Extract: Mix 10 to 20 drops in water or juice, taken daily.

Special Precautions

Blessed thistle should not be taken during pregnancy. Nursing mothers should carefully confer with an herbally oriented professional before taking blessed thistle.

BONESET (*Eupatorium perfoliatum*)

Boneset, also known as feverwort or thoroughwort, is a traditional Native American herb used in the treatment of fevers and flu. Don't be confused by the name: boneset has nothing to do with bones. Its name comes from boneset's early use in relieving the symptoms of breakbone fever, or dengue.

Infusions made from boneset are particularly effective in encouraging a sweat to break your fever. Boneset can also be used for various other conditions, such as constipation and indigestion.

Parts Used: Dried aboveground parts.

Primary Functions

▼ Boneset is a diaphoretic remedy, which means that it promotes perspiration.

▼ The most important application of boneset is in the treatment of fevers and flu.

Other Benefits

▼ Boneset may be used to treat constipation and other digestive disorders.

▼ Boneset can relieve night sweats.

▼ Boneset may be effective in the treatment of jaundice and skin diseases.

Preparation and Dosage

Boneset products are most commonly available in commercial form as capsules, extracts, and infusions.

Capsules: 4 to 10 #0 capsules up to three times daily.

Extract: Mix 10 to 40 drops in water or juice, taken daily.

Infusion: Drink 1 cup up to three times daily.

General Precautions

Boneset is a very safe herb, but normal precautions should be taken with any remedy.

BUCHU *(Barosma betulina* or *Agathosma betulina)*

Buchu, a traditional remedy of the Hottentots of Namibia and South Africa, is especially effective in the treatment of urinary and prostate disorders. Dutch and English colonists soon adopted buchu to alleviate their own similar medical problems. Benign enlargement of the prostate is a common condition in many men over the age of forty; the condition is characterized by weak urination. It should be treated as early as possible, as an enlarged prostate is often a precursor of prostate infections. Buchu is often combined with uva-ursi for this purpose.

Parts Used: Leaves.

Primary Functions

▼ Buchu is an effective treatment for benign enlargement of the prostate.

▼ Buchu is one of the most productive remedies for urinary-tract and prostate infections.

▼ Buchu is used to treat cystitis.

Other Benefits

▼ Buchu may be effective in the treatment of the early stages of diabetes.

▼ Buchu can help in cases of bed-wetting.

▼ Buchu is often recommended to treat venereal diseases.

▼ Buchu is a component of some fever remedies.

Preparation and Dosage

Buchu products are most commonly available in commercial form as capsules, tinctures, and extracts.

Capsules: 1 capsule up to three times daily.

Tincture: 1 teaspoon up to 3 times daily.

Extract: Mix 10 to 30 drops in water or juice, taken daily.

Special Precautions

If you have kidney problems, pain while urinating, or blood in your urine, do not use buchu. Buchu can irritate the kidneys, and such kidney problems require immediate medical attention.

Buchu leaves should not be boiled, as this robs the herb of its healing capabilities.

▲

BURDOCK (*Arctium lappa*)

Burdock—also known as bardane, beggar's-buttons, lappa, and thorny burr—contains chemicals called poly-acetylenes, which naturally kill bacteria and fungi. This herb is an excellent blood purifier and is rich in iron and other minerals. Burdock rids the body of toxins and promotes urine flow and perspiration. The Chinese use burdock for its calming tendencies.

Parts Used: Roots.

Primary Functions

▼ Burdock is good for blood purification; it has a cleansing effect on your blood and can rid your system of toxic conditions. Burdock's abundant iron and insulin make it an excellent tonic for your blood.

▼ Burdock can be used either internally or externally to treat skin disorders such as eczema, psoriasis, poison ivy and oak, boils, and canker sores.

Other Benefits

▼ The tendency of burdock to promote urination and perspiration can help you shed excess water weight.

▼ Burdock has a tonic effect on the stomach and kidneys.

▼ A hot burdock compress can be used to soothe the swelling of arthritis and rheumatism; it may also be helpful in dealing with hemorrhoids.

Preparation and Dosage

Burdock products are most commonly available in commercial form as capsules, extracts, and salves. A hot compress may be made by pouring hot burdock tea on a towel. (Be careful that the tea is not so hot it burns you.)

Capsules: 1 capsule up to three times daily.

Extract: Mix 10 to 25 drops of extract in water or juice, taken daily.

Salve: Apply locally as needed.

Hot Compress: Apply locally as needed.

Special Precautions

Burdock is a powerful herbal remedy and should be used with caution. It is especially important to begin use with the lowest recommended dosage; the dosage should be increased only with extreme caution. In toxic conditions, a high dosage of burdock may severely and dangerously exaggerate symptoms.

Pregnant women, nursing mothers, children, and those taking any drugs or with a specific medical condition should use burdock only under the specific guidance of a qualified herbalist or herbally oriented physician.

▲

BUTCHER'S-BROOM (*Ruscus aculeatus*)

Butcher's-broom—also known as sweet broom—is a popular European remedy for reducing leg discomfort due to poor circulation. Research conducted in France has shown that butcher's-broom contains compounds resembling steroids, and this may account for its ability to reduce inflammation. An ointment made from butcher's-broom can relieve painful hemorrhoids.

Parts Used: Leaves.

Primary Functions

▼ Butcher's-broom can relieve water retention and improve circulation; because of these properties it is used to alleviate pain in the limbs.

▼ Butcher's-broom is used in the treatment of arthritis and rheumatism.

▼ Butcher's-broom can reduce hemorrhoidal swelling.

Preparation and Dosage

Butcher's-broom products are most commonly avail-

able in commercial form as capsules, extracts, and ointments.

Capsules: 1 capsule up to three times daily.

Extract: Mix 10 to 20 drops in water or juice, taken
daily.

Ointment: Apply locally as needed.

General Precautions

Butcher's-broom is a very safe herb, but normal precautions should be taken with any remedy.

▲

CALENDULA (*Calendula officinalis*)

Calendula is a wound healer both internally and externally. It is from the same family as arnica—but calendula is
not as toxic as arnica, which cannot be taken internally.

Calendula can be used internally to treat gastritis and
duodenal ulcers. It can break your fever or alleviate menstrual cramps. Externally, this versatile herb is a soothing
remedy for burns, and it also advances the healing process
of sores and wounds. Try applying oil of calendula to relieve painful earaches.

Parts Used: Flower heads.

Primary Functions

▼ Calendula heals wounds of all kinds.

Other Benefits

▼ Calendula is an effective internal treatment for gastritis and duodenal ulcers.

▼ Calendula is taken internally to lower fevers.

▼ Internal doses of calendula can relieve the pain of menstrual cramps and ulcers.

▼ Externally, calendula stops bleeding and promotes the healing of burns and wounds.

▼ Use calendula externally to treat varicose veins.

▼ An external application of calendula salve is a valuable treatment for skin diseases such as shingles.

▼ Use calendula oil to relieve painful earaches.

Preparation and Dosage

Calendula products are most commonly available in commercial form as infusions, extracts, salves, and oils. A hot compress may be made by pouring hot calendula tea on a towel. (Be careful that the tea is not so hot it burns you.)

Infusion: 1 cup daily.

Extract: Mix 10 to 30 drops of extract in water or juice, taken daily.

Salve: Apply locally as needed.

Oil: Apply oil to a cotton swab and place it in your ear overnight.

Hot Compress: Apply locally to varicose veins, burns, and wounds.

Special Precautions

Because calendula is a uterine stimulant, it should never be used during pregnancy. Otherwise, simply exercise the normal precautions you would use with any remedy.

CASCARA SAGRADA (*Rhamnus purshiana*)

Cascara sagrada, also known as buckthorn, is one of nature's safest and gentlest laxatives. From the Latin and named by Jesuit priests, it means "holy bark" or "sacred bark." Because it is not known to be habit-forming and can be taken on a regular basis, cascara sagrada is a real boon to those who suffer from chronic constipation. It is often combined with a bulk laxative in order to be more effective.

Parts Used: Dried bark.

Primary Functions

▼ Cascara sagrada stimulates the secretions of the digestive system, making it a good all-around tonic for the gallbladder, liver, pancreas, and stomach.

▼ Cascara sagrada is a safe and mild laxative.

▼ Cascara sagrada can be used to treat cases of chronic constipation.

Other Benefits

▼ Cascara sagrada may be effective in the treatment of liver problems (such as jaundice and enlarged liver), intestinal gas, colitis, and hemorrhoids.

Preparation and Dosage

Cascara sagrada products are most commonly available in commercial form as capsules, tablets, and tinctures. The tea form of cascara sagrada is not generally taken because of its bitter taste.

Capsules: 1 capsule up to three times daily.
Tablets: 1 tablet up to three times daily.
Tincture: 1 teaspoon at bedtime.

Special Precautions

Although cascara sagrada is a safe herb and can be used on a daily basis, it is extremely important to pay attention to dosages. Begin use with the lowest dose of cascara sagrada; overdosage can cause diarrhea or cramps. The amount of cascara sagrada you take should gradually be lowered as your bowel becomes more normalized. Cascara sagrada—and any other herbs that create a laxative effect—generally should not be used during pregnancy, especially in the first trimester.

▲

CATNIP (*Nepeta cataria*)

While it drives cats crazy, catnip is most well-known for its sedative effects on the human body. Because it is such a mild herb, it is frequently recommended for hyperactive children. Often it is combined with chamomile and lemon balm to relieve nervousness.

Catnip is also effective in the treatment of colds and fevers. Europeans have long used the herb for diarrhea and bronchitis as well as for its generally calming qualities. And today, more and more Americans are coming to recognize the many versatile healing abilities of catnip.

Parts Used: Flowers and leaves.

Primary Functions

▼ Catnip has a calming, soothing influence on the nervous system. Use it to relieve stress and nervous tension.

▼ Catnip is a safe and gentle remedy for hyperactive children; but remember to check first with your pediatrician before administering any herbal remedy to your infant or child.

▼ The generally soothing nature of catnip also makes it a good cure for insomnia. Try sipping a cup of catnip tea before going to bed.

Other Benefits

▼ Catnip is used to treat colds and fevers.

▼ Catnip is an effective remedy for stress-induced diarrhea.

▼ Catnip is used to treat upper-respiratory infections such as bronchitis.

Preparation and Dosage

Catnip products are most commonly available in commercial form as capsules, tinctures, and teas.

Capsules: 1 capsule up to three times daily.

Tincture: 1 teaspoon up to three times daily.

Tea: As needed.

General Precautions

Catnip is a very safe herb, but normal precautions should be taken with any remedy.

CAYENNE (*Capsicum frutescens*)

This versatile herb found in the spice racks of many American kitchens has a variety of healing qualities. It is a mainstay of cuisines around the world—from Mexico to India to China to southern Louisiana. Cayenne is so hot and spicy that only a small pinch is necessary.

Cayenne, also known as capsicum, has many healthful qualities. It is a good digestive tonic and also benefits the heart and circulation. If you're feeling tired, it is a mild but effective pick-me-up. Cayenne is rich in vitamin C and valuable antioxidants. Externally, a cayenne poultice can ease the aches and pains of rheumatism, arthritis, and other inflammations.

Parts Used: Fruit.

Primary Functions

▼ Cayenne is a mild all-around stimulant and tonic.

Other Benefits

▼ Cayenne can improve sluggish digestion and relieve indigestion and gas.

▼ Cayenne is a good tonic for your heart and circulation. Some herbalists use cayenne to treat high blood pressure.

▼ Cayenne can stimulate your appetite; it may be helpful in treating anorexia.

▼ Cayenne is used in the treatment of colds, chills, bronchitis, and coughs. It can literally help you "sweat them out."

▼ Externally, cayenne can ease the discomfort of

rheumatism, inflammations, painful joints, and varicose veins.

Preparation and Dosage

Cayenne products are most commonly available in commercial form as capsules, teas, tinctures, and liniments. A hot compress may be made by pouring hot cayenne tea on a towel. (Be careful that the tea is not so hot it burns you.)

Capsules: 1 capsule up to three times daily.

Tea: 1 cup daily.

Tincture: 1 teaspoon up to three times daily.

Liniment: As needed.

Hot Compress: Apply locally as needed.

Special Precautions

While cayenne is generally a safe herb, it should not be used under certain conditions: Do not take cayenne if you suffer from hemorrhoids or gastrointestinal problems that have a hyperacid or ulcerative basis.

Cayenne liniment should not be used for long periods of time and should never be applied to broken skin. It should not be used on mucous membranes.

If you take cayenne internally, be careful to begin use with the lowest recommended dosage; overdosage may result in gastroenteritis or kidney damage.

CHAMOMILE (*Matricaria chamomilla*)

Chamomile is one of the most popular herbs used in the United States today. Europeans have long used chamomile as a natural herbal remedy for stress and insomnia. It is a versatile herb and can also relieve painful menstrual cramps, indigestion, and back pain. Externally, a chamomile poultice can ease the discomfort of cramps and sore muscles. Chamomile extract is used to treat skin irritations. In fact, chamomile has one of the longest and most varied lists of functions and benefits.

Parts Used: Flowers.

Primary Functions

▼ Chamomile is a safe and effective remedy to relieve everyday tension and stress.

▼ Chamomile is used to treat many of the conditions that are caused by stress, such as indigestion, a nervous stomach, and diarrhea.

▼ A weak preparation of chamomile tea is generally a safe remedy for calming irritable children and colicky or teething babies.

Other Benefits

▼ A chamomile infusion is not only soothing to your system; it can actually help you combat periodic bouts with insomnia.

▼ Chamomile can calm menstrual cramps and the tensions that accompany menopause.

▼ Chamomile eases back pain.

▼ Chamomile is used to treat kidney and bladder problems.

▼ Chamomile can help break a high fever.

▼ Chamomile is used as an inhalant for sinus infections: Make a pot of chamomile tea, put a towel over your head, and inhale.

▼ A chamomile poultice can relieve cramps, gas, swelling, and sore muscles.

▼ Chamomile extract is an effective local treatment for skin irritations.

Preparation and Dosage

Chamomile products are most commonly available in commercial form as capsules, extracts, and teas.

You can make a stronger and more effective infusion by using chamomile tea bags. Simply steep 3 chamomile tea bags in 1 covered cup of hot water for 10 minutes.

A hot compress may be made by pouring hot chamomile tea on a towel. (Be careful that the tea is not so hot it burns you.)

Capsules: 1 capsule up to three times daily.

Extract: Mix 10 to 20 drops of extract in water or juice, taken daily.

Tea: 3 to 4 cups daily.

Infusion: For insomnia, 1 cup before you go to bed.

Hot Compress: Apply locally as needed.

General Precautions

Chamomile should be used with caution by those who suffer from allergies, in case of a reaction. Otherwise, chamomile is generally a safe and soothing herb, but normal precautions, of course, should be taken with any remedy.

CHAPARRAL (*Larrea tridentata*)

Chaparral—also known as stinkweed or greasewood—is a powerful natural antibiotic. Long used by Native Americans, today even the American medical establishment has come to take a close look at chaparral. The results are controversial.

On the plus side, chaparral contains the powerful antioxidant nordihydroguaiaretic acid, or NDGA; antioxidants prevent the cell damage and abnormalities that many experts believe eventually cause cancer. A close friend of ours was told by medical doctors she would have to have her arm amputated to rid her body of cancer; instead she turned to an herbalist, who recommended a combination of chaparral, red clover, and other herbs. Today, some years later, she's alive, well, and free of cancer—and still has her arm. But chaparral should be used with caution, and only under professional supervision. In laboratory experiments long-term use of this herb has been linked to lymph and kidney problems.

Parts Used: Leaves.

Primary Functions
▼ Chaparral is a powerful natural antibiotic, making it an effective treatment for infections caused by bacteria, viruses, and parasites.

Other Benefits
▼ Because it contains the powerful antioxidant NDGA, chaparral is a popular folk treatment for cancer. There are several reports that chaparral has actually reduced cancerous tumors. If you do have cancer, consult with your

physician to see whether it is appropriate to use chaparral in conjunction with your other regular treatments.

▼ Because it includes the antioxidant NDGA, chaparral may be a way to slow the aging process. To date, however, this characteristic has only been indicated in animal studies.

▼ Chaparral is used to treat colds, flus, diarrhea, and bladder infections.

▼ Chaparral mouthwash in conjunction with regular tooth care can reduce tooth decay.

▼ Externally, chaparral is used to relieve the stiffness of arthritis.

▼ Other external uses of chaparral include the treatment of skin diseases, bruises, herpes, and eczema.

Preparation and Dosage

Chaparral products are most commonly available in commercial form as capsules, extracts, tinctures, mouthwashs, and liniments.

Capsules: 1 capsule up to three times daily.

Extract: Mix 10 to 30 drops in water or juice, taken up to three times daily.

Tincture: 1 teaspoon up to three times daily.

Mouthwash: Gargle up to three times daily.

Liniment: Apply as needed.

Special Precautions

Chaparral has wonderful healing properties—but because it is such a powerful herb, it should only be used under professional supervision. Begin use with low dosages of chaparral. Stop using the herb immediately if you develop swollen glands or difficulty in urination; consult your doctor to see why you have experienced these conditions. Pregnant and nursing women should not use chaparral, and it should not be given to children under the age of two. If you have kidney or lymph problems, do not use chaparral.

▲

CLEAVERS (*Galium aparine*)

Cleavers—also known as clivers, goose grass, and bedstraw—is a versatile and valuable plant. Its diuretic qualities increase the flow of your urine. Cleavers is also an excellent lymphatic tonic, useful in treating swollen glands, tonsillitis, and adenoid problems. In fact, cleavers is a very effective treatment for many types of inflammations. Both internally and externally, cleavers is often a good choice for relieving skin conditions such as psoriasis.

Parts Used: Aboveground parts.

Primary Functions

▼ Cleavers is one of the most powerful restorative tonics for the lymphatic system. Herbalists also use it to treat a wide variety of problems of the lymphatic system, including swollen glands, tonsillitis, and adenoid troubles.

Other Benefits

▼ The diuretic characteristics of cleavers help relieve bloating and excess water weight.

▼ Cleavers has cooling qualities that may help lower fevers.

▼ Cleavers is an effective treatment for urinary-tract infections and kidney stones.

▼ Cleavers is used in other urinary-tract conditions such as cystitis. It can ease the painful swelling of urinary and reproductive organs.

▼ Cleavers purifies the blood.

▼ Cleavers is used in the treatment of skin diseases, especially dry ones such as psoriasis.

▼ Externally, a salve made from cleavers can relieve skin rashes and burns.

Preparation and Dosage

Cleavers products are most commonly available in commercial form as capsules, extracts, tinctures, infusions, and salves.

Capsules: 5 to 10 #0 capsules up to three times daily.

Extract: ½ to 1 teaspoon up to three times daily.

Tincture: ½ to 1 teaspoon up to three times daily.

Infusion: 1 cup up to three times daily.

Salve: Apply locally as needed.

General Precautions

Cleavers is a very safe herb, but normal precautions should be taken with any remedy.

CLOVES (*Caryophyllus aromaticus*)

Cloves have been used by the Chinese for over two thousand years. In fact, Chinese citizens addressing their emperor were required to hold cloves in their mouths to conceal bad breath. Cloves are also a time-honored remedy of Ayurvedic healers in India for the treatment of respiratory and digestive disorders.

Today, cloves continue to be a popular and effective herbal remedy. Scientists have discovered that cloves are rich in the chemical eugenol, which is the source of its anesthetic and antiseptic qualities. Clove oil is an active ingredient in many over-the-counter products, such as Lavoris mouthwash.

Parts Used: Dried flowers and oil.

Primary Functions

▼ Cloves have a warming and stimulating effect upon your body.

▼ Clove oil is commonly used externally to relieve painful toothaches.

▼ A few drops of clove in warm water can relieve nausea and vomiting.

Other Benefits

▼ Cloves have anesthetic and antiseptic properties.

▼ Cloves are used to treat digestive disorders.

▼ Cloves can ease flatulence.

▼ Cloves are a restorative tonic to your digestion and circulation.

▼ Cloves are a good local antiseptic.

▼ Try a clove infusion when your hands or feet are uncomfortably cold.

▼ Cloves are often added to bitter herb remedies to make them taste better.

Preparation and Dosage

Clove products are most commonly available in commercial form as oils, infusions, extracts, and capsules.

Oil: Apply clove oil locally as needed to relieve a toothache: just pour a little on a Q-Tip or other cotton wool and put it on your sore tooth or gums.

Internally, 1 to 2 drops of clove oil in a glass of warm water can relieve nausea and vomiting; take up to three times daily.

Infusion: 1 cup up to three times daily.

Extract: 8 to 30 drops in water or juice, taken up to three times daily.

Capsules: 1 to 5 #0 capsules up to three times daily.

General Precautions

Cloves are a very safe herb, but normal precautions should be taken with any remedy.

▲

COLTSFOOT (*Tussilago farfara*)

Coltsfoot—which you may be familiar with as coughwort or horse hoof—is an expectorant and a cough suppressant that has been used from Asia to Europe for over two thousand years. Today, herbalists continue to recommend coltsfoot for a variety of respiratory problems.

But coltsfoot has become the subject of some controversy in the medical world, and so we should also exercise a little extra caution when we use it; but we still consider it safe and effective when taken in small amounts.

Parts Used: Dried flowers and leaves.

Primary Functions

▼ Coltsfoot is an excellent remedy for many respiratory problems.

▼ Coltsfoot is especially useful in relieving nonproductive dry coughs.

▼ Coltsfoot is a relaxing expectorant. It contains mucilage, a substance that tends to soothe the respiratory tract.

Other Benefits

▼ Coltsfoot is often recommended for the treatment of asthma.

▼ Many herbalists recommend coltsfoot for chronic or acute bronchitis.

▼ Coltsfoot may help in the treatment of chronic respiratory conditions such as emphysema.

▼ Coltsfoot is a good remedy for whooping cough.

▼ Externally, coltsfoot is used as a poultice for skin ulcers, due to its high zinc content.

Preparation and Dosage

Coltsfoot products are most commonly available in

commercial form as capsules, infusions, tinctures, extracts, and poultices.

Capsules: 2 to 6 #0 capsules up to three times daily.

Infusion: 1 6-ounce cup up to three times daily.

Tincture: ½ to 1 teaspoon up to three times daily.

Extract: ½ to 1 teaspoon up to three times daily.

Poultice: Mix hot water with a fresh, crushed coltsfoot leaf; put in a muslin bag and apply to the affected area.

Special Precautions

Coltsfoot contains traces of pyrrolizide alkaloids, chemicals that in large amounts can cause liver problems and cancer. But herbalists emphasize that coltsfoot has many beneficial effects when used in normal amounts. In European countries, coltsfoot continues to be a popular remedy, while American scientists remain divided on the risks versus the rewards of its use.

There are certain conditions under which it is not advisable to use coltsfoot. If you have a history of alcoholism or any other liver disease, do not use this herb. Pregnant and nursing women should not use coltsfoot, as it may damage their infants' immature livers. For the same reason, coltsfoot is not an appropriate herbal remedy for children.

Medicinal amounts of coltsfoot should be taken in consultation with a trained herbalist. If you experience side effects such as stomach upsets or diarrhea, stop taking the coltsfoot remedy and inform your herbalist or physician.

COMFREY (*Symphytum officinale*)

Comfrey, also known as knitbone, is an age-old healer that has recently become the subject of controversy in the United States. It is one of many plant substances containing chemicals that both prevent and cause cancer. On the plus side, comfrey contains antioxidant nutrients that experts believe may prevent the cell damage and abnormalities that eventually lead to cancer. And while comfrey also has toxic ingredients, it contains other constituents that induce vomiting. Therefore, if you accidentally took an inappropriately large amount of comfrey, you would vomit before it could have any toxic effect.

Comfrey has been used since ancient times for its great wound-healing qualities. It contains the chemical allantoin, which, in promoting the growth of new cells, accounts for comfrey's great healing powers. Allantoin continues to be an active ingredient in many over-the-counter and prescription skin medications, and in general the external application of comfrey has come under much less fire than its internal use.

Parts Used: Leaves and root.

Primary Functions

▼ Both internally and externally, comfrey is known to promote healing. Because of safety issues, be sure to consult with a qualified herbalist and use comfrey in appropriate amounts.

Other Benefits

▼ Because of its healing and mucilaginous qualities, comfrey is helpful in most irritated or ulcerative conditions.

▼ Comfrey is used in the treatment of wounds and sores.

▼ Comfrey can aid in the healing of broken bones. Before there was such a thing as plaster casts, comfrey paste was used to mend fractures.

▼ Because comfrey is an astringent, it can help stop bleeding.

▼ Internally, comfrey may also be useful in the treatment of digestive and lung ailments. Again, consult with your herbalist or physician before taking a comfrey remedy internally.

Preparation and Dosage

Comfrey products are most commonly available in commercial form as external ointments or skin creams. Carefully follow the directions on the label, beginning use with the lowest recommended amount.

For any internal use of comfrey, consult a qualified herbalist or an herbally oriented physician. Take note of the "Special Precautions" below.

Special Precautions

Many herbal studies indicate that the comfrey scare has been driven way out of proportion. Comfrey has actually been banned in Canada, and the United States Food and Drug Administration describes comfrey as an herb of "undefined safety." But a 1987 study concluded that the cancerous risk from drinking one cup of comfrey tea was about the same as from eating a peanut butter sandwich (peanuts may contain the naturally occurring carcinogen aflatoxin); that study, reported in *Science* magazine, was conducted by noted cancer expert Bruce Ames, chairperson of the biochemistry department at the University of California at Berkeley.

We believe that using small amounts of comfrey internally for short periods is safe. Still, there are clearly people who should steer clear of comfrey altogether, especially its internal use. If you are an alcoholic or have a history of liver disease, do not take comfrey; pregnant and nursing women should not use comfrey remedies; and comfrey should never be administered internally to children under the age of two.

Medicinal amounts of comfrey should be taken only after careful consultation with a trained professional. It is wisest to begin use with the smallest recommended dosage. Tell your herbalist or physician if you are presently taking any over-the-counter or prescription drugs, or have a specific medical condition; they can advise you of any dangerous interactions or side effects. If you experience side effects such as stomach upsets or diarrhea, stop taking the comfrey remedy and inform your herbalist or physician.

▲

CRAMP BARK (*Viburnum opulus*)

Cramp bark is an aptly named herb, for it relieves cramps and muscle spasms. It has a general tonic effect on the uterus, and it is often used to ease menstrual cramps and cramps during pregnancy. Cramp bark may be combined with other herbs, including angelica, black cohosh, black haw, false unicorn root, ginger, and valerian.

Parts Used: Dried bark.

Primary Functions
▼ Cramp bark has a general tranquilizing effect. It relaxes and soothes muscle cramps and spasms.

Other Benefits
▼ Cramp bark has a general tonic effect on the uterus and helps regulate the menstrual cycle.

▼ Cramp bark is an effective treatment for PMS and menstrual cramps.

▼ Cramp bark is used to relieve cramps during pregnancy.

▼ Cramp bark is an astringent, which means it can help control excessive bleeding during your period or in menopause.

▼ Because of its general calming and sedative qualities, cramp bark is used to treat a variety of other disorders. These include asthma, heart palpitations, hysteria, and involuntary muscle spasms.

Preparation and Dosage
Cramp bark is most commonly available in commercial form as decoctions, tinctures, and capsules.

Decoction: 1 cup up to three times daily.

Tincture: 1 teaspoon up to three times daily.

Capsules: 5 to 10 #0 capsules up to three times daily.

General Precautions
Cramp bark is a very safe herb, but normal precautions should be taken with any remedy.

CRANBERRY (*Vaccinium macrocarpon*)

Cranberry has traditionally been used by women as a natural way to prevent urinary-tract infections. A urinary-tract infection, or UTI, is a common and painful women's health problem. Cranberry juice—or capsules—seems to prevent the bacteria normally present in the urinary tract from increasing your risk of these infections.

Parts Used: Juice from the berries.

Primary Functions

▼ Cranberry may help prevent urinary-tract infections.

Preparation and Dosage

Cranberry products are most commonly available in commercial form as juices, extracts, and capsules.

Juice: Avoid sugar-laden commercial brands of cranberry juice. Instead, head to the health food store and buy a bottle of pure cranberry juice, and dilute with water if you find it too acidic or bitter. If it still tastes bitter, add a dash of maple syrup. Drink several glasses of cranberry juice each day to help prevent chronic recurrences of UTIs.

Extract: 1 teaspoon in 1 cup of water up to three times daily.

Capsules: 1 capsule up to three times daily.

General Precautions

Cranberry is generally a safe herb, but normal precautions should be taken with any remedy. If simple urinary-tract infections do not respond to herbal treatment within a few days, we advise that you should see your doctor. A course of antibiotic treatment is sometimes necessary, but there are many herbal remedies that may be tried first (for example, uva-ursi, buchu, and juniper). Cranberry products are also considered an effective way of preventing urinary-tract infections.

▲

CRANESBILL (*Geranium maculatum*)

Cranesbill is an effective remedy in many bleeding disorders. It is useful both internally and externally for a variety of problems. Taken internally, cranesbill can relieve painful and embarrassing cases of diarrhea. Externally, this herb can treat disorders ranging from hemorrhoids to burns. Cranesbill is gentle enough to use even in the very young, the elderly, and the infirm.

Parts Used: Rhizome.

Primary Functions

▼ Cranesbill has powerful astringent qualities, which makes it helpful in many cases of bleeding.

▼ Cranesbill is used internally to treat excessive bleeding during menstruation.

Other Benefits

▼ Cranesbill is used in the treatment of diarrhea, colitis, dysentery, and hemorrhoids.

▼ A cranesbill douche can relieve vaginal discharge.

▼ Cranesbill can be applied locally to treat vaginal discharge and hemorrhoids.

▼ Cranesbill can be applied externally on burns and bleeding cuts.

▼ A cranesbill gargle can be helpful for mouth and throat diseases.

Preparation and Dosage

Cranesbill is most commonly available in commercial form as capsules, decoctions, extracts, and tinctures.

Capsules: 3 to 5 #0 capsules up to three times daily.

Decoction: Simmer 1 to 2 teaspoons of cranesbill in 1 cup of water for 10 to 15 minutes. Take 1 tablespoon to 1 cup up to three times daily.

Extract: ½ to 1 teaspoon up to three times daily.

Tincture: 1 teaspoon up to three times daily.

General Precautions

Cranesbill is generally a safe herb, but normal precautions should be taken with any remedy. Remember that in any serious case of bleeding, prompt medical attention is required.

In general, douches should not be used too regularly; if the condition you are treating with a cranesbill douche persists, consult your doctor or herbalist. Never use a douche if you are pregnant.

▲

DAMIANA (*Turnera aphrodisiaca or diffusa*)

Damiana is a strengthening tonic for the nervous and hormonal systems. Traditionally, it has been used as an aphrodisiac, which may be due to an alkaloid in damiana that acts like the male hormone testosterone. Increased levels of testosterone are associated with increased sex drive in both men and women.

Small amounts of damiana may relieve anxiety and create a general sense of well-being—but care should be exercised. Excessive use of damiana may result in over-stimulation.

Parts Used: Dried leaves and stems.

Primary Functions

▼ Damiana has a strengthening tonic action on the hormonal and nervous systems.

Other Benefits

▼ Damiana has an age-old reputation as an aphrodisiac. While this cannot be scientifically verified, its alkaloids do have a testosteronelike effect. Testosterone is a male hormone.

▼ Damiana is a natural laxative.

▼ Damiana can relieve anxieties and depressions, especially when there is a sexual basis to them.

Preparation and Dosage

Damiana is most commonly available in commercial form as capsules, infusions, tinctures, and extracts.

Capsules: 1 capsule before your meal up to three times daily.

Infusion: 1 to 2 cups once daily.

Tincture: 1 teaspoon up to three times daily.

Extract: Mix 10 to 30 drops in water or juice, taken daily.

General Precautions

Damiana is a very safe herb, but normal precautions should be taken with any remedy.

▲

DANDELION (*Taraxacum officinale*)

The word dandelion comes from the French *dent-de-lion,* or "teeth of the lion," referring to the shape of the dandelion leaves. Dandelion is a valuable and nutritious herb widely used in Europe today, and has been popular in ancient cultures dating back to the ancient Chinese and Ayurvedic healers.

Animal studies have shown that dandelion leaves are a natural diuretic, which means that they increase the flow of urine. Diuretics play many valuable roles in the medical world. They are useful in relieving the bloated feeling that often accompanies PMS, and doctors often prescribe diuretics to treat high blood pressure.

The dandelion root is a helpful liver tonic. Dandelions are also packed with valuable antioxidants such as vitamin A and vitamin C; scientists believe that antioxidants can prevent the abnormal cell activity that often precedes cancer. Other studies suggest that dandelion is a digestive aid and may reduce the level of sugar in your blood.

Dandelion leaves and roots are somewhat interchangeable, but their different constituents make each more appropriate for different types of treatment.

Parts Used: Leaf and root.

Primary Functions, Dandelion Leaves

▼ Try taking a little dandelion before your period; it may help to relieve the bloating that often precedes it.

▼ High blood pressure and congestive heart failure are often treated with diuretics; but since these are both very serious conditions, ask your medical doctor before you supplement conventional medication with dandelion leaves. (Diuretics generally should not be taken on a long-term basis, since they deplete the amount of potassium in your body. But because dandelion itself is rich in potassium, it can counterbalance this effect.)

Primary Functions, Dandelion Roots

▼ Dandelion stimulates the flow of bile. This makes it a good tonic for your liver and gallbladder, and an effective treatment for liver disorders such as jaundice.

▼ Dandelion roots contain antioxidants, which may help prevent the development of cancer.

▼ Dandelion is a good digestive aid.

▼ Dandelion may reduce the amount of sugar in your body. If you have diabetes, ask your physician about incorporating dandelion into your treatment program.

Preparation and Dosage

Dandelion leaves are most commonly available in commercial form as infusions and tinctures. Dandelion root is most commonly available as decoctions and tinctures.

Infusion: 3 to 4 cups daily.

Tincture: 1 teaspoon up to three times daily.

Decoction: 3 to 4 cups daily.

General Precautions

Dandelion is a very safe herb, but normal precautions should be taken with any remedy.

▲

DEVIL'S-CLAW *(Harpagophytum procumbens)*

Devil's-claw is a traditional African and European remedy for inflammatory conditions. It is effective in the treatment of many cases of arthritis, rheumatism, and gout. Studies in Germany have compared the action of devil's-claw to cortisone and phenylbutazone; this is probably because devil's-claw contains a glycoside called harpagoside, which reduces inflammation in the joints.

Parts Used: Root.

Primary Functions

▼ The anti-inflammatory properties of devil's-claw often make it an effective treatment in cases of arthritis, rheumatism, and gout.

Other Benefits

▼ Devil's-claw is a blood purifier.

▼ Devil's-claw can expedite the elimination of uric acid from your body.

▼ Devil's-claw may be used in the treatment of liver and gallbladder problems.

Preparation and Dosage

Devil's-claw is most commonly available in commercial form as capsules, infusions, and tinctures.

Capsules: 2 to 3 #0 capsules up to three times daily.

Infusion: 1 to 2 cups daily.

Tincture: 1 teaspoon up to three times daily.

Special Precautions

Do not use devil's-claw if you are pregnant or nursing. Otherwise, devil's-claw is generally a safe herb, but normal precautions should be taken with any remedy.

DILL (*Anethum graveolens*)

Dill has been used since ancient times by civilizations ranging from the Greeks and Romans to the Egyptians and Chinese. As well as adding flavor to foods, dill is a natural preservative. It's a wonderful digestive aid and is particularly effective in cases of gas. Because dill is so mild, it is often recommended for children suffering from colic or gas.

Parts Used: Seeds.

Primary Functions

▼ Dill is an effective all-round digestive aid. It is used to treat painful stomachaches of both adults and children.

Other Benefits

▼ Dill is a good remedy for flatulence and colic.

▼ Dill tea may increase the milk flow of nursing mothers.

▼ Dill may inhibit the growth of the bacteria that cause urinary-tract infections (UTIs) in women. Many herbalists suggest adding a little dill seed oil to your bath as a preventive measure.

▼ Dill is sometimes used to treat colds, coughs, and flus.

▼ Chewing dill seeds can clear up bad breath.

Preparation and Dosage

Dill is most commonly available in commercial form as seeds, seed oils, teas, infusions, and tinctures. 1 teaspoon of dill tea is a mild but effective dose for small children suffering from colic or gas.

Seeds: Chew up to 1 teaspoon of seeds to relieve bad breath.

Seed Oil: Women can add 1 teaspoon of oil to their baths to help prevent urinary-tract infections.

Tea: Dill tea is the mildest form of dosage; it's a safe remedy for most children.

Infusion: Up to 3 cups a day.

Tincture: 1 teaspoon up to three times daily.

General Precautions

Dill is a very safe herb, but normal precautions should be taken with any remedy.

DONG QUAI (*Angelica senensis*)

Dong quai is known as the archetypal herbal remedy for women, the female ginseng. It is an ancient Chinese herb that is marvelously effective in the treatment of a wide range of women's gynecological problems. Dong quai is also a good all-around tonic for women's reproductive systems. It is a very balancing herb, and one of our personal favorites.

Parts Used: Root.

Primary Functions

▼ The tonic qualities of dong quai allow you to feel more comfortable in general.

▼ Dong quai relieves many gynecological problems, such as scanty periods, irregular periods, and the symptoms of PMS. It is particularly good in cases of nonmenstrual cramping or general weakness.

▼ Dong quai effectively relieves the symptoms of menopause, especially hot flashes.

Other Benefits

▼ Dong quai may help prevent anemia.

▼ Dong quai is used by both men and women to lower high blood pressure.

▼ Dong quai is used to treat insomnia.

▼ Dong quai may relieve constipation.

Preparation and Dosage

Dong quai is most commonly available in commercial form as capsules, tinctures, extracts, and tonics.

Capsules: 1 capsule up to three times daily.

Tincture: 1 teaspoon up to three times daily.

Extract: ½ to 1 teaspoon up to twice daily.

Tonic: In Chinese pharmacies you can find a popular and effective tonic known as Dong Quai Gin. Mix 1 tablespoon once a day in tea.

Special Precautions

When properly used, dong quai is a very safe and beneficial herb for women. However, dong quai should never be used during pregnancy. It is also not appropriate to use dong quai in cases of fibroids or excess bleeding. It is not a good idea to take dong quai if you are currently menstruating, especially if you have a heavy menstrual flow. Dong quai can aggravate loose stools or diarrhea.

▲

ECHINACEA (*Echinacea angustifolia*)

Echinacea, also known as purple coneflower, is a traditional Native American remedy with enormous immune-boosting and healing qualities. A patent-medicine maker in the nineteenth century peddled echinacea as "snake oil"; his faith in the herb was so great that he offered to visit the American Pharmaceutical Institute with a live rattlesnake, let it bite him, and cure himself with echinacea.

While echinacea has never been proven to cure the poisonous effects of rattlesnake bites, it plays many other vital roles in herbal medicine today. It is one of our favorite Western herbs, and is one of the most widely imported herbs in Europe.

Researchers have discovered that echinacea is a substance that actually strengthens your body's tissues and protects you from the attacks of invasive germs. It is best used preventively rather than curatively.

Parts Used: Leaves and root.

Primary Functions

▼ Echinacea is a good nourishing herb, an overall tonic for your body. It has slightly warming qualities. Take echinacea at the beginning of each season to ward off infection.

▼ Echinacea boosts your immune system. In a study at the University of Munich, echinacea extract increased production of infection-fighting T cells. Some preliminary research indicates that echinacea has possibilities as a cancer fighter.

▼ Echinacea contains a natural antibiotic that makes it an effective, broad-based infection fighter. It is used to treat colds, flu, bronchitis, tonsillitis, tuberculosis, and meningitis.

Other Benefits

▼ Echinacea can help heal wounds.

▼ Echinacea may be used in the treatment of cuts, burns, eczema, and psoriasis because of its blood-cleansing abilities.

▼ When echinacea is taken with traditional antifungal creams, studies have shown that women are less likely to experience the recurrence of a vaginal yeast infection.

▼ Echinacea may have an anti-inflammatory effect and has been successfully used in treating some cases of arthritis.

Preparation and Dosage

Echinacea products are most commonly available in commercial form as capsules, tinctures, decoctions, and extracts.

Capsules: 1 capsule up to three times daily.

Tincture: 1 teaspoon up to three times daily.

Decoction: 1 cup up to three times daily.

Extract: Mix 15 to 30 drops in water or juice, taken up to four times daily.

General Precautions

Echinacea causes a small tingling sensation on your tongue—but this is not a bad thing. In fact, if you do not experience this sensation, the herb may not be effective. Echinacea is generally a very safe herb; side effects are rare, even after taking large doses.

ELDER (*Sambucus nigra*)

Elder is an old Gypsy remedy for colds and flus. Today it is also used for related problems in the upper respiratory tract, including hay fever and sinusitis. Some recommend elder in the treatment of arthritis and rheumatism. Externally, elder is appropriate for a wide host of problems, including bruises, burns, and rashes. Elder can also be used cosmetically to clear the skin and reduce wrinkles.

Parts Used: Berries, flowers, and leaves.

Primary Functions

▼ Elder is used in the treatment of colds and flus. To this purpose it is often combined with other herbs, such as peppermint, yarrow, or ginger. Drink 1 cup of one of these mixtures, wrap yourself up in plenty of warm covers, and try to sweat your cold out or break your fever.

▼ Elder can be helpful in relieving upper-respiratory ailments, such as hay fever and sinusitis.

Other Benefits

▼ Elder is used to treat arthritic and rheumatic problems.

▼ Elder is a natural laxative.

▼ Externally, elder acts as a salve for minor skin problems, such as bruises, wounds, burns, and rashes.

▼ Elder is used externally to clear up wrinkles.

Preparation and Dosage

Elder products are most commonly available in commercial form as capsules, infusions, tinctures, and extracts. Elder is often combined with other herbs in commercial preparations; take care to follow the directions on any commercial remedy.

Capsules: 5 #0 capsules up to three times daily.

Infusion: 1 cup up to three times daily.

Tincture: 1 teaspoon up to three times daily.

Extract: ½ to 1 teaspoon up to three times daily.

General Precautions

Elder is generally a safe herb, but normal precautions should be taken with any remedy.

▲

ELECAMPANE (*Inula helenium*)

Elecampane—also known as horseheal, scabwort, velvet dock, and wild sunflower—is an ancient remedy that many herbalists continue to recommend for a wide variety of respiratory problems. Chinese and Indian Ayurvedic doctors used elecampane to treat bronchitis and asthma, which are still its major uses. In addition, the Greeks and Romans praised the great digestive healing powers of elecampane.

Parts Used: Root.

Primary Functions

▼ Elecampane is an excellent remedy for respiratory problems such as asthma, bronchitis, tuberculosis, emphysema, and whooping cough.

▼ Elecampane promotes expectoration. It is unique in

that it is good for tight as well as productive coughs. This is due to its combination of relaxing and stimulating qualities.

Other Benefits

▼ Elecampane contains a chemical that can help prevent intestinal parasites and expel them from your body. You might want to tuck some elecampane in your suitcase on your next Caribbean vacation.

▼ Elecampane is a good digestive tonic.

▼ Elecampane stimulates the appetite.

Preparation and Dosage

Elecampane products are most commonly available in commercial form as capsules, decoctions, and tinctures.

Capsules: 5 #0 capsules up to two times daily.

Decoction: 1 to 2 teaspoons at a time, up to twice daily.

Tincture: ¼ to ½ teaspoon up to three times daily.

Special Precautions

Diabetics should not use elecampane, as it may raise blood sugar. Otherwise, elecampane is a very safe herb, but normal precautions should be taken with any remedy.

▲

EPHEDRA (*Ephedra sinica*)

Ephedra is thought to be the world's oldest herbal remedy. It has been used since ancient times to treat asthma and upper-respiratory infections.

Ephedra was first cited as a medicinal plant in the Vedas, or ancient scriptures of India. In China, where ephedra is known as *ma huang,* herbologists have used ephedra to treat asthma for more than five thousand years. Early Mormon settlers in the United States made "squaw tea" from ephedra to treat asthma.

Two alkaloids that are naturally present in ephedra are used today in a number of over-the-counter medications for asthma, bronchitis, and allergies. The alkaloids have evidently opposite effects on the body, but the overall action is that of balance and benefit.

The alkaloids of ephedra may also be spotted as constituents of diet formulas. But buyer beware! Diet pills are not any magic answer to your weight problem. A sensible diet and exercise program recommended by your doctor is the best way to lose weight and keep it off.

Parts Used: Aboveground stems.

Primary Functions

▼ Ephedra is useful in treating the symptoms of asthma, allergies, and upper-respiratory infections, such as stuffy nose and watery eyes.

▼ Ephedra may also be used in cases of bronchitis, emphysema, hay fever, and whooping cough.

Other Benefits

▼ Ephedra may relieve headaches, rheumatism, and arthritis.

▼ Due to its unique combination of constituents, ephedra has a slight stimulating effect.

▼ Ephedra may help to bring on menstruation.

Preparation and Dosage

Ephedra products are most commonly available in commercial form as capsules, decoctions, and tinctures. Ephedra is a powerful herb and should only be used for short periods of time.

Capsules: 5 to 10 #0 capsules up to three times daily.

Decoction: 1 cup up to three times daily.

Tincture: 1 teaspoon up to three times daily.

Special Precautions

Pregnant and nursing women should not use ephedra; it may cause miscarriage. Parents should consult with their pediatrician before administering ephedra to children.

One of the active constituents of ephedra, ephedrine, is a strong stimulant to the central nervous system. Ephedra is on the list of banned substances of the United States Olympic Committee.

Some people use ephedra to lose weight. We do not recommend ephedra for this purpose. Regular aerobic exercise and a low-fat, high-fiber diet are the long-term solutions to any weight problem.

Side effects of ephedrine include high blood pressure and heart palpitations. It should not be used by anyone who has high blood pressure, heart disease, thyroid disease, glaucoma, or diabetes without professional supervision.

Do not take more than the recommended dose stated on the labels of ephedra remedies. Begin any treatment with ephedra remedies with the lowest recommended dosage, and take ephedra only for limited periods of time.

While taking ephedra you may experience insomnia, nervousness, and dry mouth. Talk to a qualified professional about any side effects you may experience. If you should experience an upset stomach while taking ephedra, try taking your recommended dosage at mealtime.

If you are presently taking any over-the-counter or prescription drugs, or have a specific medical condition, it is especially important to consult an herbally oriented physician before using ephedra. Ephedra can have dangerous interactions with medications that raise blood pressure.

▲

EUCALYPTUS (*Eucalyptus globulus*)

Eucalyptus—also known as Australian gum, blue gum, and gum tree—has been approved by the United States Food and Drug Administration as a cold and flu remedy. The eucalyptus tree is native to Australia, although it has now been planted in countries around the world.

Eucalyptus leaves contain the chemical eucalyptol, which gives this herb its unique healing qualities and pleasant aroma. Eucalyptol is an active ingredient in many over-the-counter products, such as Vicks VapoRub, Dristan decongestant, and Sine-Off.

Parts Used: Leaves.

Primary Functions
▼ Eucalyptus is an effective treatment for upper-respiratory ailments, notably colds, flu, and bronchitis.

▼ Eucalyptus is a good expectorant. Simply inhaling it loosens the phlegm in your chest.

Other Benefits

▼ Eucalyptus is a powerful natural antiseptic. It may be useful in treating minor cuts or scrapes.

▼ Use a eucalyptus ointment to relieve painful arthritis and rheumatism.

▼ According to a report in *Science News,* eucalyptol may help you get rid of cockroaches.

Preparation and Dosage

Eucalyptus products are most commonly available in commercial form as liniments, oils, and leaves.

Liniment: Apply as needed according to package directions.

Oil: Apply 1 to 2 drops to minor scrapes and wounds. As an inhalant for colds and flu, put a few drops of the essential oil into hot water and breathe deeply. Rub a little oil directly on your skin to relieve arthritic pain.

Leaves: Wrap a handful of eucalyptus leaves in cheesecloth for a refreshing herbal bath.

Special Precautions

Eucalyptus oil should not be taken internally; as little as 1 teaspoon of eucalyptus oil taken internally can prove fatal. Some commercial preparations—such as cough drops and salves—contain nontoxic amounts of eucalyptus. The external application of eucalyptus is generally considered safe and helpful.

EVENING PRIMROSE (*Oenothera biennis*)

Evening primrose, also known as sundrops, is an old Native American herb. The oil of evening primrose has a high content of gammalinolenic acid (GLA), which is converted by your body into prostaglandins; these are fatty acids that act much like hormones, producing a wide range of effects on your body. Evening primrose is useful in treating a wide variety of ailments, ranging from PMS to hypertension to inflammatory conditions.

Parts Used: Leaves and oil from seed.

Primary Functions
▼ Evening primrose can reduce the symptoms of PMS, such as headaches, painful breasts, irritability, and bloating.

Other Benefits
▼ Evening primrose may be used to treat hypertension; but since hypertension is a serious condition, remember to consult with your physician before incorporating evening primrose into your medical regimen.

▼ Evening primrose can relieve anxiety.

▼ Evening primrose is a traditional remedy for arthritis.

▼ Evening primrose is used to treat eczema and is considered safe enough for use in small children.

Preparation and Dosage
Evening primrose products are most commonly available in commercial form as capsules.

Capsules: 1 250-milligram capsule up to three times daily.

Special Precautions

Evening primrose should not be taken by pregnant women, as prostaglandins may cause uterine contractions.

Otherwise, evening primrose is generally a safe herb; simply take the normal precautions that you would with any remedy.

▲

EYEBRIGHT (*Euphrasia officinalis*)

Eyebright has been used since the Middle Ages to treat eye ailments. This herb is especially beneficial in treating inflammations of the eyes and sinuses. It is cooling to the blood.

Eyebright is a good alternative to the commercial eyedrops regularly used to eliminate redness. Over time, commercial eyedrops can actually worsen this problem; they work by constricting blood vessels, which with each successive use will enlarge in less time.

Parts Used: Dried aerial parts.

Primary Functions

▼ Eyebright is useful as a nurturing tonic in promoting general eye health, and as a cure for a variety of problems that may affect the eye.

Other Benefits

▼ Eyebright can soothe the inflamed, itchy, irritated eyes and sinuses that accompany colds and allergies.

▼ Eyebright can be used to treat conjunctivitis.

▼ Eyebright may relieve eyestrain.

▼ Eyewashs made of eyebright in combination with other herbs, such as goldenseal, fennel, or bayberry, can relieve irritated and swollen eyes.

Preparation and Dosage

Eyebright products are most commonly available in commercial form as capsules and eyewashs.

Capsules: 1 capsule up to three times daily.

Eyewash: Follow the dosage schedule on the label. An eyewash can generally be used every 4 hours.

General Precautions

Eyebright is generally a safe herb, but normal precautions should be taken with any remedy.

▲

FALSE UNICORN ROOT *(Chamaelirium luteum)*

False unicorn root, also known as helonias root, is one of the best supportive tonics for women's reproductive systems. The active constituents of false unicorn root, one of our favorite herbs, are actually precursors of estrogen. This old Native American remedy is also used to treat a variety of women's reproductive and gynecological problems. False unicorn root may often be combined with other herbs, such as cramp bark.

Parts Used: Root.

Primary Functions

▼ The principal use of false unicorn root is to regulate women's menstrual cycles. It is especially helpful in cases of painful or irregular menstruation. Results don't take place overnight: a three-month course of treatment is usually necessary.

Other Benefits

▼ False unicorn root has a good general tonic effect on women's reproductive systems.

▼ False unicorn root is used to treat infertility in women and impotence in men.

▼ False unicorn root is sometimes used by pregnant women to prevent a threatened miscarriage and to ease morning sickness. If you are pregnant, always consult your obstetrician or midwife before taking any remedy.

Preparation and Dosage

False unicorn root is most commonly available in commercial form as decoctions, tinctures, and capsules.

Decoction: 1 cup up to three times daily.

Tincture: 1 teaspoon up to three times daily.

Capsules: 2 to 5 #0 capsules up to three times daily.

General Precautions

False unicorn root is generally a safe herb, but normal precautions should be taken with any remedy.

▲

FENNEL (*Foeniculum vulgare*)

Fennel, also known as finocchio or carosella, was a favorite remedy of the ancient Greeks and Romans. In our own country, the Puritans used fennel as a digestive aid, and it is still used in this way. Fennel is a versatile herb helpful in a wide variety of ailments, such as gynecological problems, rheumatism, and conjunctivitis.

Parts Used: Seeds.

Primary Functions
▼ Fennel soothes the digestive tract.
▼ Fennel is an effective remedy for flatulence (gas).
▼ Fennel relieves cramps and indigestion.

Other Benefits
▼ Fennel is used in the treatment of coughs and colds.
▼ A very weak infusion of fennel may ease the discomfort of your colicky infant; but check first with a professional herbalist or herbally oriented pediatrician.
▼ If you are a nursing mother, fennel may increase the flow of your breast milk. (Again, first consult with your qualified professional.)

▼ Fennel may be used to bring on a menstrual period.

▼ Some women take fennel to ease the discomforts experienced during menopause.

▼ Fennel oil may be applied locally to ease rheumatic pains.

▼ A fennel infusion may be used to treat conjunctivitis.

▼ Chewing fennel seeds relieves bad breath.

Preparation and Dosage

Fennel products are most commonly available in commercial form as seeds, infusions, tinctures, and oils.

Seeds: Chew up to ¹/₂ ounce of the seeds each day. You can toast or roast the seeds and they're very tasty.

Infusion: Up to 3 cups daily.

Tincture: ¹/₂ to 1 teaspoon up to three times daily.

Oil: Apply locally as needed. *Never* take the oil internally; it may cause nausea and vomiting.

General Precautions

Fennel is a very safe herb, but normal precautions should be taken with any remedy.

FENUGREEK (*Trigonella foenumgraecum*)

The use of fenugreek dates back to the ancient Greeks and Romans. Today, fenugreek is used by some non-pregnant women to bring on a late period. According to some studies, it may also help reduce high levels of cholesterol and blood sugar. Many herbalists use fenugreek to treat colds, coughs, and sore throats. Applied locally, fenugreek may help wounds heal and ease the ache of arthritis.

Parts Used: Seeds.

Primary Functions

▼ Fenugreek contains a chemical similar to the female hormone estrogen; taking it may help bring on a late menstrual period.

▼ Fenugreek may relieve sore throats, bronchitis, colds, and coughs.

Other Benefits

▼ Research has shown that fenugreek reduces blood cholesterol levels in animals; although this is promising, the results have not yet been confirmed in humans.

▼ Fenugreek has been shown to reduce blood sugar levels in animal studies; if you are diabetic, talk to your doctor about possibly incorporating fenugreek into your regular medical regimen.

▼ Nursing mothers may want to consult a qualified professional about using fenugreek to increase their breast milk. Fenugreek is generally considered a safe herb for this purpose.

▼ Externally, fenugreek may help heal wounds and sores.

▼ The local application of fenugreek may reduce the inflammation and thus ease the pain of arthritis.

Preparation and Dosage

Fenugreek products are most commonly available in commercial form as decoctions, tinctures, and poultices.

Decoction: Up to 3 cups daily. Add other herbs, such as aniseed or peppermint, to improve the flavor.

Tincture: ¼ to ½ teaspoon up to three times daily.

Poultice: Mix hot water with ground fenugreek seeds; put in a muslin bag and apply to the affected area.

Special Precautions

Pregnant women should not use fenugreek, since it is a uterine stimulant. Otherwise, fenugreek is generally a safe herb; simply take the normal precautions that you would with any remedy.

FEVERFEW (*Tanacetum parthenium*)

Feverfew—also known as featherfew and midsummer daisy—is a wonder herb for migraine sufferers. Don't be misled by the name: feverfew does not reduce fevers. But, in 1988, the prestigious British medical journal *Lancet* verified its ability to cut down significantly on both the rate of occurrence and the severity of migraine headaches. Often chewing a few feverfew leaves each day (today you can also opt for a feverfew capsule or pill) helps migraine sufferers for whom years of standard medical treatments did nothing.

Parts Used: Leaves.

Primary Functions

▼ Feverfew is a wonderful remedy for those who suffer from chronic migraine headaches. In many cases occurrences of headaches are lessened or even prevented altogether. When migraine headaches do occur, they are generally less severe, with less nausea, vomiting, and pain.

Other Benefits

▼ Feverfew may help reduce high blood pressure; but since hypertension is a serious condition, remember to consult with your physician before incorporating feverfew into your medical regimen.

▼ Feverfew is a digestive aid. If you experience indigestion, try taking it after meals.

▼ Feverfew may relieve menstrual cramps.

▼ Feverfew may alleviate anxiety.

Preparation and Dosage

Feverfew products are most commonly available in commercial form as capsules or pills. Some herbal shops also offer the leaves, which you can chew on.

Capsules: 1 capsule up to three times daily.

Pills: 1 pill up to three times daily.

Special Precautions

Feverfew is generally a safe herb. However, it's important to exercise certain precautions in its use. Pregnant women should not take feverfew. If you have a history of blood clotting, consult your physician before taking feverfew. Chewing on the leaves of feverfew sometimes causes mouth sores. If this happens to you, take capsules or pills instead.

▲

FO-TI (*Polygonum multiflorum*)

Fo-ti, known as *ho shou wu* in China, is a longevity tonic. It gives energy and strength, and is especially rejuvenating to the elderly. Fo-ti is a good overall restorative tonic for your blood, kidneys, and liver. It is said to improve the digestion and increase fertility, and has a reputation as an aphrodisiac. The Chinese believe that fo-ti can even keep your hair from going gray. A popular brand of fo-ti sold in Chinese herb stores is an alcoholic preparation called Shou Wu Chih.

Parts Used: Root.

Primary Functions

▼ Fo-ti is a longevity tonic. It may prevent premature aging or slow the aging process.

▼ Fo-ti restores energy and strength.

▼ Fo-ti is good for your blood, kidneys, and liver.

Other Benefits

▼ Fo-ti may be useful in the treatment of hypoglycemia, diabetes, and deficiency diseases.

▼ Fo-ti is a digestive aid.

▼ Fo-ti may increase fertility and act as an aphrodisiac.

Preparation and Dosage

Fo-ti products are most commonly available in commercial form as capsules, decoctions, and tinctures. Fo-ti pills and tonics are also widely available in Chinese pharmacies.

Capsules: 1 capsule up to three times daily.
Decoction: 2 ounces two to four times daily.
Tincture: 1 teaspoon up to three times daily.

General Precautions

Fo-ti is generally a safe herb, but normal precautions should be taken with any remedy.

▲

GARLIC (*Allium sativum*)

Garlic is among the world's oldest and most effective herbal remedies. Ancient healers from Greece to India used garlic to treat a wide range of ailments. The Egyptian slaves who built the pyramids were given a daily ration of garlic to prevent disease and promote strength; according to one tale, society's first strike took place when garlic became scarce and the slaves were denied their rations.

More recently, garlic was the remedy of choice for treating wounded soldiers during World War I. Although penicillin was discovered in 1928 and antibiotics replaced garlic after then, when the Russian army ran out of penicillin in World War II they turned again to garlic. After that, garlic was nicknamed the Russian penicillin.

Parts Used: Bulb.

Primary Functions

▼ Garlic reduces the level of cholesterol and plaque in your heart's arteries. Take it to improve your overall heart health.

▼ Raw garlic contains a natural antibiotic that makes it an effective, broad-based infection fighter. When garlic is chewed or crushed, this powerful antibiotic chemical is released. A combination of crushed raw garlic and honey may be just the thing to cure a sore throat.

Other Benefits

▼ Garlic is an excellent overall tonic for your body. Take it daily to strengthen your digestive and respiratory systems. Garlic also protects your body from disease.

▼ Garlic may help in the treatment of colds, flu, bronchitis, whooping cough, food poisoning, blood diseases, bowel infections, and women's bladder and vaginal yeast infections.

▼ Studies suggest that garlic may prevent stomach and other types of cancer.

▼ Exciting new research indicates that garlic may help in the treatment of AIDS.

▼ Garlic regulates your blood pressure so effectively that it is used to treat both high and low blood pressure.

▼ Garlic has an anticlotting action that decreases your risk of heart attack and stroke. If you already suffer from a clotting disorder, consult with your doctor before taking medicinal amounts of garlic.

▼ Garlic reduces the level of sugar in your blood; if

you are diabetic, talk to your doctor about possibly incorporating garlic into your regular medical regimen.

▼ Garlic is a digestive aid. Use it to relieve gas and indigestion.

▼ Garlic may help eliminate lead from your blood. Lead can cause serious· brain damage, especially in children.

▼ Externally, garlic is used to treat ringworm and other skin parasites.

▼ Rub garlic oil into your skin to soothe aching muscles.

▼ A few drops of garlic oil in your ear will help clear up an earache.

Preparation and Dosage

Garlic products are most commonly available in commercial form as fresh cloves, capsules, tinctures, and oils.

Fresh Cloves: It's the volatile oil of the raw cloves of garlic that gives them their antibiotic effect. When you take away their smell, the cloves lose their antibiotic effect. Cooked garlic loses its active ingredients. To get rid of a cold: crush 1 clove of raw garlic in 1 teaspoon of honey and eat it. Then cover yourself up and just sweat it out. If raw garlic tastes too strong for you, try one of the following preparations instead.

Capsules: 1 capsule up to three times daily.

Tincture: ½ to 1 teaspoon up to four times daily.

Oil: To make garlic oil, chop four to six cloves of garlic and heat (do not fry) in a pint of olive oil. This process extracts its active ingredients for safe and effective use.

For colds, flu, and fever, take 1 teaspoon of garlic oil in

lemon juice or water each hour. For earaches, put 2 to 3 drops in the ear up to twice daily. For skin parasites, warts, or muscular aches and pains, apply locally as needed.

General Precautions

Garlic is a safe and healthy herb. Still, all good things in moderation. There's a trick about working with raw cloves of garlic: squeezing lemon over your hands usually eliminates the odor. For garlic breath, try chewing a few aniseed or fennel seeds to freshen your mouth.

GENTIAN (*Gentiana lutea*)

Gentian is an excellent bitter tonic that stimulates the digestion. Ancient Egyptians, Greeks, and Romans all used gentian for a variety of ailments. Gentian encourages the production of saliva, stomach acid, and bile. Gentian can perk up a sluggish appetite and relieve nausea and flatulence (gas). Chinese studies indicate that gentian may also be helpful in the treatment of inflammatory conditions such as arthritis.

We recommend packing a one-ounce bottle of gentian tincture when you travel to countries where dysentery is common. A couple of drops on your tongue before each meal will make your stomach very acidic. Pathogens that could otherwise cause stomach problems are headed off at the pass, killed by the acid in your stomach.

Parts Used: Root.

Primary Functions

▼ Gentian is a supportive and nurturing bitter tonic for the digestion. It is also used to treat a variety of digestive disorders.

Other Benefits

▼ Gentian stimulates the appetite.

▼ Gentian relieves a variety of digestive disorders, such as nausea, vomiting, heartburn, and flatulence.

▼ Gentian may help prevent food poisoning.

▼ Gentian has anti-inflammatory properties that may make it useful in the treatment of arthritis.

Preparation and Dosage

Gentian products are most commonly available in commercial form as decoctions and tinctures.

Decoction: 1 cup before meals.

Tincture: Up to 1 teaspoon before meals.

Special Precautions

While gentain is an excellent digestive herb, it should be avoided during pregnancy. Although it has not been proven, gentian has a reputation for promoting menstruation.

GINGER (*Zingiber officinale*)

Mothers have traditionally given their children a warm glass of ginger ale—usually with the admonition to sip it slowly—to relieve nausea and vomiting. It turns out we've been on the right track. Ginger is a good digestive aid and has an antispasmodic, antinausea action. A study in the respected British journal *Lancet* showed that ginger was actually more effective than Dramamine in preventing motion sickness. Ginger is also used in the treatment of colds, flu, and a variety of other ailments.

Parts Used: Root.

Primary Functions

▼ Ginger is used to relieve nausea and indigestion, and to calm an upset stomach.

▼ Ginger may help prevent motion sickness.

▼ A glass of ginger ale is a safe remedy for pregnant women who suffer from morning sickness. Or you may try a few drops of ginger tincture on your tongue to relieve a queasy feeling.

▼ Drink cups of ginger tea to help you sweat out a fever.

Other Benefits

▼ Patients undergoing chemotherapy often experience nausea; ginger may help to alleviate it.

▼ A very weak ginger preparation may be used in infants to relieve the symptoms of colic.

▼ Ginger is used in the treatment of colds, bronchitis, and flus. In one Chinese study, ginger was shown to help kill a flu virus.

▼ Ginger's antispasmodic qualities also make it valuable in the relief of menstrual cramps.

▼ Ginger may be useful in the treatment of arthritis.

▼ Ginger can reduce the level of cholesterol in your blood, according to a study in *The New England Journal of Medicine*. Lower cholesterol means a healthier heart.

▼ Externally, ginger may soothe sore muscles and skin inflammations such as mumps.

Preparation and Dosage

Ginger products are most commonly available in commercial form as capsules, infusions, and tinctures. To relieve nausea, you might also try simply sipping a 12-ounce glass of ginger ale.

Capsules: 1 capsule up to three times daily.

Infusion: To make a fresh infusion shave 1 teaspoon of fresh ginger from a ginger root, and pour 1 cup of hot water over it. Cover and let it steep for 10 minutes. Drink up to 3 cups daily.

Tincture: 1 teaspoon up to three times daily.

General Precautions

Ginger is a very safe herb, but normal precautions should be taken with any remedy. If you experience heartburn as a side effect when taking ginger to relieve motion sickness, cut down on your dosage or try another remedy.

GINKGO (*Ginkgo biloba*)

Ginkgo, also known as the maidenhair tree, is one of the oldest trees on earth. It is also one of the most widely prescribed herbal remedies in Europe, embraced by herbalists and medical doctors alike. Ginkgo has a unique ability to inhibit a process called platelet activity factor (PAF). PAF plays a major role in many of your body's processes, such as blood flow and blood clots. By blocking PAF, ginkgo exhibits tremendous healing possibilities.

Ginkgo trees can live three to four thousand years. In an appropriate parallel, ginkgo may also be a valuable healing aid to the elderly. As ginkgo improves blood flow to all parts of the body, for example, there may be decreased risk of the type of stroke that occurs when blood flow to the brain is blocked; heart attack prevention (by reducing the blood clots that cause them); and stimulation of memory and reaction time (again by increasing blood flow to the brain).

Parts Used: Leaves and nut.

Primary Functions

▼ Ginkgo may be effective in preventing or treating many of the conditions that increasingly affect us as we age.

▼ Ginkgo improves blood circulation.

▼ Ginkgo may decrease your risk of stroke.

▼ In one study, ginkgo was shown to improve memory and reaction time. It may prove to be a treatment for Alzheimer's disease.

Other Benefits

▼ Ginkgo may help prevent heart attacks.

▼ Ginkgo has been used to treat circulation problems associated with diabetes. It is said to improve blood flow in the legs.

▼ Ginkgo may be useful in the treatment of asthma.

▼ In a French study, ginkgo was successfully used to treat tinnitus (chronic ringing in the ears).

▼ In another study, ginkgo relieved the chronic dizziness of a group of people suffering from vertigo.

▼ Exciting new research indicates that ginkgo may help your body accept transplanted organs.

Preparation and Dosage

Ginkgo products are most commonly available in commercial form as capsules, tablets, and tinctures.

Capsules: 1 40-milligram capsule up to three times daily.

Tablets: 1 40-milligram tablet up to three times daily.

Tincture: 1/2 to 1 teaspoon up to three times daily.

Special Precautions

Because of ginkgo's PAF-inhibiting quality, ginkgo is not an appropriate herbal remedy for those with blood clotting disorders. However, it is generally considered a safe herb.

The only indicated use of ginkgo for children is in the treatment of asthma.

It is essential to carefully follow the dosage directions on commercial ginkgo remedies. Large quantities of ginkgo may cause side effects such as nausea, diarrhea, or irritability. If the dosage on the label is stated in terms of a range, begin use with the lowest dosage.

▲

Women and Ginseng

While ginsengs are generally considered to be male tonics, women recovering from disease or debility can use them on a short-term basis. Ginseng can be used by women for up to three months during convalescence.

▲

GINSENG, AMERICAN *(Panax quinquefolium)*

American ginseng, which is primarily grown in Wisconsin, was traditionally used by Native Americans to treat nausea and vomiting. Somewhat milder and less stimulating than Asian ginseng, American ginseng is now used around the world. It is the ginseng that is most appropriate for women to use before menopause; Asian and Siberian ginseng are more appropriate for men.

Both Asian and American ginseng contain chemicals called ginsenosides. While no one fully understands how they work, advocates of both types of ginseng believe that ginsenosides make this herb the classic overall tonic for your body.

American ginseng, like Asian and Siberian, can help you deal more effectively with both emotional and physical stress. It can counteract the effects of stress and fatigue on your body. Ginseng may increase your resistance to disease by stimulating your immune system. And today, some American athletes take ginseng to improve their performances, as Russian and Asian athletes have long done.

Parts Used: Root.

Primary Functions

▼ Ginseng is an excellent overall tonic for your body.

▼ Ginseng allows you to cope more efficiently with both emotional and physical stress.

▼ Ginseng may counteract fatigue.

▼ Ginseng can boost your immune system, and therefore increase your resistance to disease.

▼ Ginseng may improve physical stamina.

▼ Ginseng stimulates the appetite, which can be especially useful for the elderly.

Other Benefits

▼ Ginseng may improve your memory.

▼ Several studies have indicated that ginseng reduces your total blood cholesterol level.

▼ Ginseng has an anticlotting action that may reduce your risk of heart attack.

▼ Ginseng may be used by diabetics to reduce blood sugar levels. Since diabetes is a serious disease, consult with a qualified professional before incorporating ginseng into your regular treatment regimen.

▼ Ginseng is often recommended by herbalists for the treatment of respiratory problems.

▼ Ginseng may enhance liver function.

Preparation and Dosage

American ginseng products are most commonly available in commercial form as capsules, decoctions, and tinctures.

Capsules: 1 capsule up to three times daily.

Decoction: 1 cup up to twice daily.

Tincture: ½ to 1 teaspoon up to three times daily.

General Precautions

Because all types of ginseng are popular herbal remedies, they have been subject to adulteration. To avoid buying phony ginseng, carefully read the label of the product you buy. Look for products made by reputable companies and made from the whole, unprocessed root.

Although side effects of American ginseng are rare, there have been some reports of insomnia and allergic symptoms while taking this herb. If you experience these reactions, stop using ginseng. American ginseng is not an appropriate remedy for children.

GINSENG, ASIAN (*Panax ginseng*)

Asian ginseng is an ancient herbal remedy highly revered in China and Korea. It is more powerful and stimulating than American ginseng. Like American ginseng, Asian ginseng contains chemicals called ginsenosides, which researchers believe make this herb the classic overall tonic to relieve emotional and physical stress in men. Ginseng stimulates the immune system and can therefore increase your resistance to disease. Asian athletes have traditionally used ginseng to enhance their performances.

Asian ginseng is primarily a tonic for men, as it contains precursors of testosterone. But it is also appropriate for women to use for short periods during convalescence, and is a menopausal herb. The equivalent Chinese herb for women is dong quai.

Parts Used: Root.

Primary Functions

▼ Ginseng is an excellent overall tonic for men's bodies.

▼ Ginseng is used in the treatment of general states of weakness and exhaustion.

▼ Ginseng is an adaptogenic herb. That is, it helps you adapt to emotional and physical stress.

▼ Ginseng stimulates the production of white blood cells, which boosts your immune system and increases your resistance to disease.

▼ Ginseng may improve physical stamina. This may account for its traditional use as an aphrodisiac.

▼ Ginseng may counteract the symptoms of menopause in women.

▼ Ginseng stimulates the appetite, which can be especially useful for the elderly.

Other Benefits

▼ Ginseng may increase your concentration and enhance your memory.

▼ Ginseng has been shown to reduce cholesterol.

▼ Ginseng has an anticlotting action that may reduce your risk of heart attack.

▼ Ginseng may reduce blood sugar levels. If you are diabetic, talk with your physician or a qualified herbal professional about taking ginseng.

▼ Ginseng is often recommended by herbalists for the treatment of respiratory problems.

▼ Ginseng may improve liver function.

▼ In Chinese studies, Asian ginseng has been shown to be useful in the treatment of stomach cancer.

Preparation and Dosage

Asian ginseng products are most commonly available in commercial form as capsules, decoctions, and powders. Because of the stimulating effect of ginseng, young people should not take it for more than three weeks at a time. Under the careful supervision of a qualified herbal practitioner, older people sometimes take smaller amounts of this herb for extended periods in order to restore vitality.

Capsules: 1 capsule up to three times daily.

Decoction: 1 cup up to three times daily.

Powder: 5 to 10 grams in liquid daily.

Special Precautions

Because Asian ginseng is more stimulating than American ginseng, avoid taking it too close to bedtime. If you find that it makes you feel nervous or anxious, reduce your dosage or discontinue taking the herb. Do not take it with caffeine. People with high blood pressure should not take Asian ginseng.

Because Asian ginseng may increase estrogen levels in women, it is usually not an appropriate remedy for women until menopause. At menopause, Asian ginseng can be a natural alternative to hormone replacement therapy.

Be sure that the Asian ginseng you buy is the real thing. Adulterated or diluted ginseng sometimes finds its way into the market because of the extreme popularity of this herb. Buy Asian ginseng made by well-known and respected herbal companies.

Asian ginseng is not an appropriate remedy for children. If you are presently taking any over-the-counter or prescription drugs or have a specific medical condition (such as high blood pressure), speak to an herbalist or herbally oriented physician before taking Asian ginseng; they can advise you of any dangerous interactions or side effects.

▲

GINSENG, SIBERIAN *(Eleutherococcus senticosus)*

Siberian ginseng is not true ginseng, but its chemical components have so many of the same actions that it is known as ginseng. It is even more stimulating than Asian ginseng, and so should be used with care. Like Asian ginseng, Siberian ginseng is a tonic for men, and is not recommended for use by women until after menopause, except during brief periods of convalescence.

Siberian ginseng contains chemicals called eleutherosides, which act in many ways like the ginsenosides in true ginseng. Like Asian ginseng, Siberian ginseng is an overall tonic to relieve emotional and physical stress in men. Siberian ginseng also increases resistance to disease, improves vitality and stamina, and may be helpful in the treatment of cardiovascular disorders and diabetes. It is often used by Russian athletes.

Parts Used: Root.

Primary Functions

▼ Ginseng is a stimulating tonic for men.

▼ Ginseng is used in the treatment of general states of weakness and exhaustion.

▼ Ginseng increases mental alertness and relieves physical stress.

▼ Ginseng can increase your resistance to diseases such as infections and colds.

▼ Ginseng may improve physical stamina.

▼ Ginseng may counteract many of the symptoms of aging.

Other Benefits

▼ Ginseng is used in the treatment of heart disease, since it helps reduce blood cholesterol.

▼ Ginseng may help in the treatment of diabetes, as it may reduce blood sugar levels. Consult with your physician or a qualified professional before taking ginseng.

Preparation and Dosage

Siberian ginseng products are most commonly available in commercial form as capsules and extracts. Because of its highly stimulating effect, Siberian ginseng should only be used for a month at a time.

Capsules: 1 capsule up to three times daily.

Extract: 5 to 10 drops in warm liquid daily.

Tincture: ½ to 1 teaspoon up to three times daily.

Special Precautions

Because Siberian ginseng can be stimulating, do not take it close to bedtime. If you find that it makes you feel nervous or anxious, reduce your dosage or discontinue taking the herb. People with high blood pressure should consult with their physician before using Siberian ginseng.

Siberian ginseng is not an appropriate remedy for women or children for prolonged use. If you are presently taking any over-the-counter or prescription drugs, or have a specific medical condition (such as high blood pressure), speak to an herbalist or herbally oriented physician before taking Siberian ginseng; they can advise you of any dangerous interactions or side effects.

GOAT'S RUE (*Galega officinalis*)

Goat's rue is a bitter herb that helps regulate sugar levels in your body; it contains the alkaloid galegine, which is responsible for this action. Because of this function, goat's rue may be a useful complementary treatment for adult-onset diabetes. However, remember that diabetes is a serious disease; herbal treatment should be taken only after consulting with your physician.

Parts Used: Dried aboveground parts.

Primary Functions

▼ Goat's rue can reduce your blood sugar level. It may be used under professional supervision to supplement regular medical treatment of diabetes.

Other Benefits

▼ Goat's rue may increase milk production by stimulating the mammary glands. If you are a nursing mother, consult a qualified professional about using goat's rue.

Preparation and Dosage

Goat's rue products are most commonly available in commercial form as infusions and tinctures.

Infusion: Up to 2 cups daily.

Tincture: 1/2 to 1 teaspoon up to three times daily.

General Precautions

Goat's rue can be a very helpful herb. But since it may have a very powerful effect on your body, it's a good idea to consult a qualified professional before using goat's rue.

Goat's rue is not a replacement for the regular medical treatment of diabetes, yet it can be a very valuable supplement to that treatment. Talk to an herbally oriented physician to see if goat's rue is right for you.

Goat's rue is not an appropriate remedy for children. If you are both pregnant and diabetic, you should exercise extreme caution in the use of any remedy, and no remedy whatsoever should be taken without very extensive communication with your doctor.

If you are a nursing mother seeking to increase your milk production, consult with a qualified professional before using goat's rue to accomplish this.

GOLDENSEAL (*Hydrastis canadensis*)

Goldenseal, also known as yellow root, is such a useful and versatile herb that in the nineteenth century it became known as the "poor man's ginseng." Goldenseal contains two alkaloids, berberine and hydrastine, that are responsible for many of its valuable nurturing and healing abilities.

Goldenseal is a natural antibiotic and an immune-system booster. It is valuable in the treatment of a wide variety of symptoms and ailments, such as diarrhea, digestive problems, adults' ear infections, and respiratory problems such as those associated with bronchitis, the flu, and hay fever.

Parts Used: Root.

Primary Functions

▼ Goldenseal is a powerful natural antibiotic that can be used to treat many conditions.

▼ Goldenseal is soothing to the intestines. In many cases, it has proved to be an effective treatment for digestive problems such as colitis and gastritis.

▼ Goldenseal is used in the treatment of upper-respiratory problems, such as bronchitis and hay fever.

Other Benefits

▼ Goldenseal can boost your immune system by increasing white blood cell production.

▼ Goldenseal kills many of the bacteria that cause diarrhea.

▼ Goldenseal may help clear up adults' ear infections. Milder herbal remedies are more appropriate for infants and children.

▼ Goldenseal may relieve uncomfortable flu symptoms.

▼ Goldenseal has a bitter action that stimulates the appetite.

▼ Goldenseal may reduce heavy menstrual flow.

▼ Externally, goldenseal can be helpful in some cases of athlete's foot, conjunctivitis, earache, eczema, and itching.

Preparation and Dosage

Goldenseal products are most commonly available in commercial form as capsules, infusions, and tinctures.

Goldenseal has a bitter taste, so you may want to mix it with honey or lemon.

Capsules: 2 to 5 #0 capsules up to three times daily.

Infusion: Up to 2 cups daily.

Tincture: ½ to 1 teaspoon up to three times daily.

Special Precautions

Goldenseal is generally a safe and valuable herb, but normal precautions should be taken with any remedy.

Goldenseal should never be taken during pregnancy, since it may stimulate muscles in the uterus.

Goldenseal should also not be taken if you have high blood pressure, heart disease, diabetes, or glaucoma, because one of its active constituents, hydrastine, may raise blood pressure.

GOTU KOLA (*Centella asiatica*)

Gotu kola—also known as sheep rot, Indian pennywort, water pennywort, and marsh pennywort—is an ancient herbal remedy prized alike by Chinese physicians and Indian Ayurvedic healers. In these cultures it is still thought to promote longevity, similar in its rejuvenating powers to fo-ti and ginseng.

More recently, a British study showed gotu kola to be an effective treatment for leprosy, or Hansen's disease. This may be because gotu kola contains the chemical asiaticoside, which enables the immune system to destroy bacteria. Gotu kola can also improve leg circulation, and externally it may accelerate the healing of wounds and relieve inflammatory skin diseases such as psoriasis.

Parts Used: Leaves.

Primary Functions

▼ Gotu kola is a relaxant and nervous-system restorative.

▼ Gotu kola may have rejuvenating properties that promote longevity.

Other Benefits

▼ Gotu kola may promote blood circulation in the lower limbs.

▼ Studies have shown that gotu kola hastens the healing of wounds and burns and minimizes scarring.

▼ Gotu kola may be useful in the treatment of skin diseases ranging from psoriasis to Hansen's disease.

▼ Gotu kola may help relieve varicose veins.

▼ Gotu kola may be a blood purifier and may aid in the healing of blood diseases.

Preparation and Dosage

Gotu kola products are most commonly available in commercial form as capsules, infusions, and tinctures. For external use, make a compress by pouring a hot gotu kola infusion on a towel. (Make sure that the infusion is not so hot it burns you.)

Capsules: Take as directed.

Infusion: Up to 2 cups daily.

Tincture: 1/2 to 1 teaspoon up to three times daily.
Compress: Apply locally as needed.

General Precautions

Gotu kola is generally a safe herb, but normal precautions should be taken with any remedy.

▲

HAWTHORN (*Crataegus oxyacantha*)

Hawthorn—also known as maybloom or mayflower—is one of the best herbal tonics for the heart and the circulatory system. Hawthorn also helps your body adapt to physical, emotional, and environmental stress.

Hawthorn contains the active constituents saponins and glycosides, which can normalize heart function by either stimulating or depressing it, depending on your heart's need. Hawthorn balances any heart problem: if you have high blood pressure, hawthorn lowers it; if you have low blood pressure, hawthorn raises it.

Hawthorn can be used safely for long periods of time to treat heart conditions ranging from heart failure to high blood pressure. Because heart problems are serious and can be life-threatening, consult a qualified professional before using hawthorn.

Hawthorn has also been used traditionally in Chinese medicine for its digestive qualities. Hawthorn is one of our favorite herbs.

Parts Used: Berries.

Primary Functions

▼ Hawthorn is an excellent tonic remedy for the heart.

Other Benefits

▼ Hawthorn can be used to treat heart failure or weakness.

▼ Hawthorn helps normalize heart palpitations.

▼ Hawthorn may aid in the lowering of high blood pressure.

▼ Hawthorn may help open coronary arteries, which makes it helpful in cases of atherosclerosis.

▼ Hawthorn can ease the chest pains of angina.

▼ Chinese herbalists prize hawthorn for its digestive qualities.

Preparation and Dosage

Hawthorn products are most commonly available in commercial form as infusions or tinctures.

Infusion: Up to 2 cups daily.

Tincture: ¹/₂ to 1 teaspoon up to three times daily.

General Precautions

Hawthorn is generally a safe and effective remedy. However, if you have serious medical—especially heart—problems, see a qualified professional.

Hawthorn is not an appropriate remedy for children, or for pregnant or nursing women.

While hawthorn can safely be taken for extended periods of time, your dosage should be closely monitored by a qualified practitioner. If you are presently taking any over-the-counter or prescription drugs or have a specific medical condition, speak to an herbalist or herbally oriented physician before taking hawthorn; they can advise you of any dangerous interactions or side effects.

▲

HOPS (*Humulus lupulus*)

Hops, also known as humulus, has a sedative effect on the central nervous system and is also used as a digestive aid. Chemicals in hops are believed to kill bacteria and may therefore help prevent infection. A sedative chemical, 2-methyl-3-butene-2-ol, was discovered in hops in 1983, and lends credence to its long reputation as a tranquilizer. Hops may be particularly effective in easing the tension accompanied by indigestion.

Parts Used: Flower strobiles.

Primary Functions
▼ Hops is a sedative and a digestive aid.

Other Benefits
▼ Hops can be useful in treating some cases of insomnia.
▼ Hops may help fight infection.

Preparation and Dosage
Hops products are most commonly available in commercial form as capsules, infusions, and tinctures.

Capsules: 5 to 10 #0 capsules up to three times daily.

Infusion: 1 warm cup before bedtime to relax and get a good night's sleep.

Tincture: ½ to 1 teaspoon up to three times daily.

Special Precautions

Hops should not be taken if you suffer from depression. Hops is otherwise a safe herb, but normal precautions should be taken with any remedy. If the dosage on the label is stated in terms of a range, begin use with the lowest dosage.

Anecdotal evidence suggests that hops may bring on menstruation. While there is no proof of this, pregnant women should exercise caution and avoid using hops. Nursing women should take hops only after conferring with their obstetrician or midwife. Hops is generally an inappropriate herb for children.

▲

HORSE CHESTNUT *(Aesculus hippocastanum)*

Horse chestnut has a strengthening and toning effect on the circulatory system. In particular, this herb is an excellent supportive remedy for veins and hemorrhoids. It can be used both internally and externally.

Part Used: Fruit.

Primary Functions
▼ Horse chestnut can reduce the swelling of varicose veins and hemorrhoids.

Other Benefits
▼ Horse chestnut may also be useful in the treatment of other circulatory disorders, such as phlebitis.

Preparation and Dosage
Horse chestnut products are most commonly available as infusions, tinctures, and lotion.

Infusion: 1 cup up to three times daily.

Tincture: 1 teaspoon up to three times daily

Lotion: Apply as needed according to package directions.

General Precautions
Horse chestnut is a very safe herb, but normal precautions should be taken with any remedy.

▲

HORSETAIL (*Equisetum arvense*)

Horsetail—also known as bottlebrush, pewterwort, scouring rush, and shave grass—was used by ancient Roman and Chinese physicians to treat wounds. Its active constituent—silica—makes it one of the most effective herbal remedies for urinary-tract problems (such as cystitis), benign enlargement of the prostate, and gout.

Horsetail is composed of almost 10 percent silica, which has valuable astringent, or binding, qualities. This is the highest amount of silica in almost any plant. Horsetail also has diuretic qualities. Diuretics increase the flow of urine, but also deplete the body of potassium. Remember to eat plenty of potassium-rich foods such as bananas when you take a diuretic.

Parts Used: Stems.

Primary Functions

▼ Because of its diuretic qualities, horsetail is a good internal remedy for urinary and prostate disorders.

Other Benefits

▼ Horsetail is used externally to heal wounds.

▼ Horsetail may be useful in easing painful joint conditions such as arthritis.

Preparation and Dosage

Horsetail products are most commonly available in commercial form as capsules, infusions, tinctures, and poultices. Horsetail should only be used for brief periods of time.

Capsules: 5 to 10 #0 capsules up to three times daily.

Infusion: Up to 2 cups daily.

Tincture: 1/2 to 1 teaspoon up to three times daily.

Poultice: To relieve joint pain, soak a cotton towel in a hot horsetail infusion and place on inflamed area.

Special Precautions

While horsetail is a wonderful herb with many healing qualities, it is not right for everyone. Horsetail contains selenium, which in large amounts may cause birth defects, and should be avoided by pregnant women.

▲

JUNIPER (*Juniperus communis*)

Juniper, also called geneva, is probably best known as the basis of gin, which the Dutch invented using juniper in the seventeenth century. In the Middle Ages, people planted juniper trees outside their homes to scare away witches. Its smoke was said to prevent the bubonic plague and leprosy.

Today, juniper is valued by herbalists for its antiseptic and diuretic qualities. In fact, juniper is an ingredient in a number of over-the-counter diuretics. Diuretics increase the flow of urine, but also deplete the body of potassium. Remember to eat plenty of potassium-rich foods such as bananas when you take a diuretic.

Parts Used: Berries.

Primary Functions
▼ Juniper is an excellent remedy for urethral and bladder infections, as well as the gout. (It is *not* appropriate for kidney pain.)

Other Benefits

▼ Juniper is recommended by some herbalists for the treatment of occasional flare-ups of inflamed conditions such as arthritis. It is not, however, an appropriate remedy for chronic arthritis.

▼ Because juniper is a diuretic, it may be helpful in treating a variety of symptoms and ailments. These include high blood pressure and congestive heart failure.

Preparation and Dosage

Juniper products are most commonly available in commercial form as capsules, infusions, and tinctures. Juniper should only be used for six weeks at a time, because over time it can irritate the kidneys.

Capsules: Up to 10 #0 capsules up to three times daily.

Infusion: Up to 2 cups daily.

Tincture: ½ to 1 teaspoon up to three times daily.

Special Precautions

Juniper should not be taken if you are or suspect you might be pregnant. It is also an inappropriate remedy if you have any history of kidney damage. Avoid taking juniper if you have hay fever.

Juniper should not be taken for more than six weeks at a time, because it may irritate your kidneys. Begin use with the lowest recommended dosages of juniper. Beware of symptoms of overdose, such as diarrhea, kidney pain, blood in the urine, and high blood pressure.

If you are presently taking any over-the-counter or prescription drugs, or have a specific medical condition, consult an herbally oriented physician before using juniper.

LADY'S MANTLE *(Alchemilla vulgaris and xanthochlora)*

Lady's mantle is a popular European herb for the relief of all types of bleeding. As you might suspect from the name, it's an especially good remedy for women. As well as tempering excessive menstrual bleeding, lady's mantle eases menstrual cramps and alleviates many of the symptoms of menopause. Its astringent qualities also make lady's mantle a good remedy for diarrhea.

Parts Used: Leaves and stems.

Primary Functions

▼ Lady's mantle has a role in reducing all kinds of bleeding, especially excessive bleeding associated with menstruation.

Other Benefits

▼ Lady's mantle may reduce menstrual pains.

▼ Lady's mantle can relieve many symptoms of menopause.

▼ Lady's mantle is used in the treatment of diarrhea.

▼ Gargling with lady's mantle may relieve laryngitis.

▼ A mouthwash of lady's mantle can aid in the healing of sores in the mouth.

Preparation and Dosage

Lady's mantle products are most commonly available in commercial form as infusions, tinctures, and mouthwash.

Infusion: Up to 3 cups daily.

Tincture: ½ to 1 teaspoon up to three times daily.

Mouthwash: As needed.

Special Precautions

Lady's mantle should not be used if you are pregnant. It is otherwise a a safe herb, but normal precautions should be taken with any remedy.

▲

LAVENDER (*Lavandula officinalis*)

Lavender is probably best known as a perfume, but this herb also has many valuable medicinal qualities. It can help relieve your tension headaches and lift you out of a mild depression. Lavender's gentle action can help you slip into a soothing and natural sleep. Gently rub lavender oil on your temples when you have a headache, or use it locally to relieve arthritic pain.

Parts Used: Flowers.

Primary Functions

▼ Lavender has a nurturing tonic effect on your nervous system, which makes it valuable in treating ailments such as stress-related headaches and depression.

Other Benefits

▼ Lavender may be useful in soothing nervous conditions.

▼ Lavender can ease cases of exhaustion.

Preparation and Dosage

Lavender products are most commonly available in commercial form as an infusions or oils. The oil should *not* be taken internally.

Infusion: Up to 3 cups daily.

Oil: Rub the oil on your skin or pour some in your bath.

General Precautions

Lavender is a very safe herb, but normal precautions should be taken with any remedy.

▲

LEMON BALM (*Melissa officinalis*)

Lemon balm is a gentle herb with a mintlike flavor. Rub the fresh leaves together and smell—delicious! And lemon balm is so mild that it can be used to treat infants' colic. Lemon balm is particularly suitable for many types of children's disorders, such as colds and flus. Lemon balm relieves anxiety and tension, and is an excellent, pleasant-tasting digestive relaxant for people of all ages.

Parts Used: Leaves.

Primary Functions

▼ Lemon balm may be used to treat digestive disorders and the symptoms of cold and flu. It is a particularly gentle and relaxing herb, and children enjoy its minty taste.

Other Benefits

▼ Lemon balm is a digestive relaxant. Use it in cases of indigestion or flatulence (gas).

▼ Lemon balm tea can be taken by nursing mothers of colicky babies. The herb may soothe their irritability and restlessness as it is passed on to them through mother's milk.

▼ Lemon balm can ease nervous tension. Drink a cup of lemon balm tea after a busy day or to relax before you go to bed at night.

▼ Lemon balm may help relieve depression.

▼ Lemon balm is used to treat colds and fevers.

▼ Externally, lemon balm ointment may relieve the symptoms of herpes simplex.

Preparation and Dosage

Lemon balm products are most commonly available in commercial form as teas, tinctures, and ointments. To make tea for an adult, use 3 teaspoons of the dried herb to 1 cup of hot water. Children's tea can be made with 1 ounce of dried lemon balm; if you like, you can also sweeten it with honey.

Tea: 3 to 4 cups daily. The tea is mild enough to take on a very frequent basis.

Tincture: 1/2 to 1 teaspoon up to three times daily.

Ointment: Use locally as needed to relieve the symptoms of herpes simplex.

General Precautions

Lemon balm is an especially safe and gentle herb. Because it is so mild, it is often used in children's remedies.

▲

LICORICE (*Glycyrrhiza glabra*)

Licorice can help suppress coughs, heal ulcers, and treat inflammations. A Japanese study is even investigating the cancer-fighting possibilities of licorice.

In Chinese medicine, licorice is called the great unifier: it brings out the primary functions of other herbs it is combined with. As a result of this synergistic effect on herbal combinations, all the herbs work together more effectively.

While licorice has many valuable healing qualities, it should be used in moderation. Large amounts of licorice can result in unpleasant and even dangerous side effects, and licorice is not the right herb for everyone. (See the "Special Precautions" below.)

Parts Used: Root.

Primary Functions

▼ Licorice may help suppress coughs.

▼ Licorice is a good remedy for lung problems such as colds and flu.

▼ Licorice provides relief for certain kinds of ulcers.

In one study, GA, the chemical in licorice, proved as effective as the ulcer drug Tagamet in treating duodenal ulcers.

▼ Because licorice supports the adrenal function, it has anti-inflammatory properties that make it useful in cases of arthritis.

▼ Licorice is a soothing relaxant with expectorant qualities. It is often added to more bitter formulas to make them more palatable.

Other Benefits

▼ Licorice may help prevent infection.

▼ Licorice cream may ease skin inflammations such as eczema.

▼ Licorice may help heal the painful cold sores of herpes simplex.

▼ Licorice is a mild laxative.

▼ Licorice may be a good liver tonic.

▼ Research is being done on the potential cancer-fighting qualities of licorice.

Preparation and Dosage

Licorice products are most commonly available in commercial form as capsules, decoctions, tinctures, extracts, syrups, or creams. Licorice is a powerful herb and should only be used for brief periods of time.

Capsules: 1 capsule up to three times daily.

Decoction: Up to 2 cups daily.

Tincture: ½ to 1 teaspoon up to twice daily.

Extract: ½ to 1 teaspoon up to three times daily.

Syrup: 1 to 3 teaspoons as needed.
Cream: Apply locally as needed.

Special Precautions

Licorice has wonderful healing properties, but it is not right for everyone. Since licorice may result in an increase in blood pressure, it is not appropriate if you have a history of hypertension, diabetes, glaucoma, stroke, or heart disease. Pregnant and nursing women should not take licorice remedies.

Because licorice is such a powerful herb, low dosages should be used and only for brief periods of time. Consult your pediatrician before administering any licorice remedy to a child. Stop using the herb immediately if you experience side effects such as headaches, bloating (watch out for swollen ankles), or lethargy.

LOBELIA (*Lobelia inflata*)

North American Indians used to smoke lobelia instead of tobacco. Lobelia is a nurturing and supportive tonic for the lungs, applicable to a wide variety of upper-respiratory ailments. Lobelia is particularly helpful in the treatment of asthma and bronchitis and a valuable addition to all cough remedies—and its expectorant qualities make it especially good for spasmodic productive coughs.

Different dosages of lobelia have different effects. (See "Preparation and Dosage" below.) Unfortunately, many people find it hard to stomach the taste of lobelia. Sometimes adding licorice to a lobelia formula helps the taste. Other times similar lung tonics, such as elecampane, can be substituted for lobelia.

Parts Used: Leaves and seeds.

Primary Functions

▼ Lobelia is primarily a lung tonic. It is useful in the treatment of a range of upper-respiratory ailments, especially asthma. Bronchitis and coughs may also be relieved with lobelia.

▼ A tincture of lobelia and cramp bark can help reduce nicotine addiction. Give it a shot if you're trying to quit smoking.

Other Benefits

▼ Lobelia may help relieve fevers associated with upper-respiratory conditions.

▼ Lobelia may relieve cramps.

▼ Lobelia is sometimes used, under the guidance of a qualified professional, for the treatment of hysteria and convulsions.

▼ Lobelia may be helpful in cases of food poisoning. Keep in mind, however, that food poisoning is a severe and possibly life-threatening condition. Consult a qualified professional before taking any action.

▼ Externally, lobelia may be useful in the treatment of arthritis, bruises, insect bites, poison ivy, ringworm, and sprains.

Preparation and Dosage

Because different dosages of lobelia have very different actions, it's important to pay special attention to this category.

One half to one teaspoon of lobelia tincture has a sedative effect, may help you quit smoking, and is used to treat respiratory problems. Lobelia can be taken up to three times a day for these conditions.

A tablespoon or so of lobelia tincture acts as an emetic: that is, it makes you vomit. If you find yourself in a situation where you don't have access to an emergency room, lobelia may be helpful in cases of food poisoning. But keep in mind that food poisoning is a serious condition. Contact your doctor or local Poison Control Center before taking any action. (Keep these numbers posted on your telephone or refrigerator, especially if you have children.)

Special Precautions

Lobelia contains a nicotinelike alkaloid called lobeline, which has prompted some concern among researchers. But actually, this can work to your advantage when you are using a lobelia combination to quit smoking.

While lobelia is generally a safe herb, normal precautions should be taken with any herbal remedy. Pay special attention to dosages of lobelia, as different dosages have different effects.

Pregnant and nursing women should take lobelia only after conferring with their obstetrician or midwife. Parents should consult with their pediatrician before administering any herbal remedy to children.

If you are presently taking any over-the-counter or prescription drugs, or have a specific medical condition, speak to an herbalist or herbally oriented physician before taking lobelia; they can advise you of any dangerous interactions or side effects.

▲

MARIGOLD (*Calendula officinalis*)

Marigold is a valuable herb both externally and internally. It's a handy first-aid treatment for minor wounds and burns, and marigold ointment is an effective remedy for varicose veins. Marigold is often a component of eyewash for conjunctivitis.

On an internal basis, try taking marigold to relieve indigestion. Marigold is soothing to ulcers and can help regulate menstrual periods.

Parts Used: Flower petals.

Primary Functions

▼ Internally, marigold may aid in the relief of indigestion and ulcers.

▼ Applied externally, marigold is an especially effective herb for treating local skin disorders.

Other Benefits

▼ Marigold may be taken internally to relieve gallbladder problems.

▼ Marigold is used internally to help regulate menstrual periods.

▼ Marigold may be applied to minor wounds, burns, bruises, and strains.

▼ You can use marigold ointment locally to relieve painful varicose veins and hemorrhoids.

▼ Marigold is often included in commercial eyewashs for conjunctivitis.

Preparation and Dosage

Marigold products are most commonly available in commercial form as infusions, tinctures, and ointments.

Infusion: Up to 3 cups daily.

Tincture: 1 teaspoon up to three times daily.

Ointment: Apply locally as needed.

Special Precautions

Since marigold has a reputation of bringing on delayed periods, it should not be used internally if you are or suspect you may be pregnant.

Otherwise, marigold is generally a safe herb, but normal precautions should be taken with any remedy.

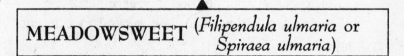

MEADOWSWEET *(Filipendula ulmaria or Spiraea ulmaria)*

In 1853 German scientists developed the first aspirin from an extract of meadowsweet. Meadowsweet, also known as bridewort and queen of the meadow, is a fragrant herb that contains an aspirinlike chemical called salicin.

Salicin is the precursor of aspirin: it relieves pain, reduces fever, and has anti-inflammatory qualities.

Today, many people use meadowsweet as a mild alternative to aspirin. It is often helpful in reducing fever and relieving pain, and it does not cause the stomach upset that many people experience when they take aspirin. In fact, far from irritating your tummy, meadowsweet itself is an excellent digestive aid.

Parts Used: Leaves and flower tops.

Primary Functions

▼ Meadowsweet is a good remedy for colds, flu, and low-grade fevers.

▼ Meadowsweet may relieve the pain of arthritis and rheumatism.

▼ Meadowsweet is recommended for a variety of digestive disorders, such as nausea and heartburn.

▼ Meadowsweet is a gentle remedy for diarrhea in children.

Other Benefits

▼ Meadowsweet may be used to relieve headaches.

▼ Meadowsweet is used to ease general muscle and joint pain.

▼ Meadowsweet may ease menstrual cramps.

Preparation and Dosage

Meadowsweet products are most commonly available in commercial form as infusions and tinctures.

Infusion: Up to 3 cups daily.

Tincture: 1 teaspoon up to three times daily.

General Precautions

Meadowsweet is generally a safe herb, but normal precautions should be taken with any remedy. Although meadowsweet is considered mild enough to treat children's diarrhea, parents should consult with a qualified professional before administering any remedy to their young children.

Meadowsweet is not an appropriate remedy for children under two, or for children under the age of sixteen who are suffering from a cold, fever, flu, or chicken pox. This is because meadowsweet's relative, aspirin, has been linked with Reye Syndrome, a potentially fatal condition associated with children's fevers. This is not to say that there has ever been any evidence that meadowsweet itself has any link with Reye Syndrome—but it is better to err on the side of caution and avoid giving this herb to feverish children.

▲

MILK THISTLE (*Silybum marianum*)

Milk thistle, also known as St.-Mary's-thistle, is an excellent liver tonic. The liver plays a vital role in detoxifying the poisons (such as alcohol and pollutants) that enter our bloodstream. Milk thistle contains a substance called silymarin that increases the flow of all-important bile from the liver, whose primary function is to break down poisons and fats.

Parts Used: Seeds.

Primary Functions

▼ Milk thistle is a nurturing and supportive liver tonic.

▼ Milk thistle is considered a safe herb to increase the flow of breast milk in nursing mothers.

Other Benefits

▼ Milk thistle may be a helpful addition to the medical treatment of those suffering from liver disease.

▼ Milk thistle may counteract the impact of irritants such as exposure to secondary smoking and other pollutants.

Preparation and Dosage

Milk thistle products are most commonly available in commercial form as capsules, infusions, and tinctures.

Capsules: 1 capsule up to three times daily.

Infusion: Up to 3 cups daily.

Tincture: 1 teaspoon up to three times daily.

General Precautions

Milk thistle is a very safe herb, but normal precautions should be taken with any remedy.

MOTHERWORT (*Leonurus cardiaca*)

True to its Latin description as *cardiaca,* motherwort stabilizes the heart. This herb is a useful addition to any strengthening and supportive heart tonic. German research has noted that motherwort has tranquilizing qualities similar to valerian; it's helpful in easing heart palpitations and other conditions due to nervous tension.

Motherwort contains a chemical called leonurine, which is a uterine stimulant. Motherwort should not be used during pregnancy—but 1 warm cup of motherwort tea can bring on suppressed menstruation in women.

Parts Used: Leaves, flowers, and stems.

Primary Functions

▼ Motherwort is an excellent heart tonic.

▼ Motherwort can reduce the hot flashes of menopause.

▼ Motherwort has sedative qualities.

▼ Motherwort promotes menstruation.

Other Benefits

▼ Motherwort can relieve heart conditions such as palpitations and tachycardia.

▼ Motherwort eases all sorts of nervous tension.

▼ Motherwort may be an effective treatment for insomnia.

▼ Motherwort is used to relieve the symptoms of menopause and PMS.

▼ Motherwort may be taken during painful menstrual periods, especially those associated with anxiety.

Preparation and Dosage

Motherwort products are most commonly available in commercial form as extracts, infusions, or tinctures. Since motherwort has a somewhat bitter flavor, mix it with honey, lemon, or maple syrup.

Extract: Mix 10 to 15 drops in warm water up to three times daily.

Infusion: Up to 2 cups daily.

Tincture: ½ to 1 teaspoon up to twice daily.

Special Precautions

Motherwort is generally a safe herb. However, it should never be used during pregnancy, since it is a uterine stimulant. Those with clotting disorders or high blood pressure should use this herb with caution.

▲

MULLEIN (*Verbascum thapsus*)

Mullein—also known as Aaron's rod, candlewick, feltwort, lady's foxglove, lungwort, shepherd's club, torch, and velvet dock—is a supportive remedy for all types of respiratory ailments. Native Americans once inhaled smoked mullein leaves to ease congestion.

German studies have revealed that mullein contains mucilage, a substance that swells and soothes respiratory irritations as it absorbs water. Coughs, colds, and sore throats are all relieved by remedies that contain mullein. Mullein is also useful in the treatment of diarrhea and hemorrhoids.

Parts Used: Flowers, leaves, and roots.

Primary Functions

▼ Mullein is an excellent remedy for all sorts of respiratory problems, such as asthma, bronchitis, congestion, coughs, colds, hay fever, and sore throats.

Other Benefits

▼ Mullein may be a helpful auxiliary treatment for emphysema. Since emphysema is a serious disease, consult first with your doctor before supplementing regular medical care.

▼ Mullein compresses are good for hemorrhoids.

▼ Mullein and mullein oil may help relieve diarrhea.

▼ Mullein may relieve swollen glands.

Preparation and Dosage

Mullein is most commonly available in commercial form as extracts, infusions, oils, tinctures, or compresses. Mullein remedies should be used for about two weeks at a time. If your symptoms do not improve by then, consult your doctor.

Extract: Mix 25 to 40 drops in warm water up to twice daily.

Infusion: Up to 3 cups daily.

Oil: Put 2 or 3 drops of warmed mullein oil in your ear overnight to relieve an ear infection.

Tincture: ½ to 1 teaspoon up to three times daily.

Compress: Locally apply a compress of mullein infusion to relieve painful hemorrhoids.

General Precautions

Mullein is a very safe herb, but normal precautions should be taken with any remedy.

▲

| MYRRH (*Commiphora myrrha*) |

Myrrh has been prized by herbalists for thousands of years. The Bible mentions myrrh as one of three precious gifts presented to the baby Jesus by the wise men. Ancient Greeks and Romans used myrrh to treat wounds and digestive problems.

Modern Chinese researchers have discovered that myrrh can help kill the bacteria that lead to tooth decay and gum disease. Myrrh stimulates the production of white blood cells, which also fight infection.

Myrrh is a prominent ingredient in natural mouthwashes and toothpastes available in many health food stores. You can also dab a little tincture of myrrh on a cotton swab and use it to relieve mild tooth pain. Serious toothaches, of course, require a trip to the dentist.

Parts Used: Gum resin.

Primary Functions

▼ Myrrh is a good local antiseptic for the treatment of wounds.

▼ Myrrh is especially good for mouth and gum infections.

▼ Myrrh is good for all sorts of mouth problems, such as bleeding gums, canker sores, gingivitis, and bad breath.

Other Benefits

▼ Myrrh is an effective treatment for digestive and intestinal disorders.

▼ Myrrh is useful for the treatment of all throat diseases.

▼ Myrrh may relieve chronic diarrhea.

▼ Some early studies have indicated that myrrh may reduce blood cholesterol.

Preparation and Dosage

Myrrh products are most commonly available in commercial form as capsules, infusions, tinctures, and mouthwashs or gargles. You can mask the somewhat bitter flavor of myrrh infusions by mixing them with honey, lemon, or maple syrup.

Capsules: 2 to 6 #0 capsules up to three times daily.

Infusion: Up to 2 cups daily.

Tincture: ¼ to 1 teaspoon up to three times daily.

Mouthwash or Gargle: As needed.

General Precautions

Myrrh is generally a safe herb, but normal precautions should be taken with any remedy. Since myrrh has a traditional (although unproven) reputation of bringing on delayed menstrual periods, it should not be used internally if you are or suspect you may be pregnant.

OATS (*Avena sativa*)

Oats are an excellent remedy for the nervous system. They are soothing in cases of stress, tension, and depression. Since digestive problems are sometimes connected to the nervous system, oats may also be taken for irritated digestive conditions such as ulcers and gastroenteritis.

Oat straw contains high levels of silicic acid, which makes it an effective treatment for many skin diseases—especially those associated with nervous conditions. Try using an external oat-straw preparation to relieve shingles and herpes.

Parts Used: Seeds and straw.

Primary Functions

▼ Oats are one of the best supportive and nurturing tonics for the nervous system.

▼ Oats can be used to alleviate digestive problems associated with stress and tension.

▼ Oats can be applied externally to relieve skin diseases, especially those with a nervous basis.

Other Benefits

▼ Use oats to treat cases of depression and exhaustion.

▼ Oats may relieve some of the symptoms of menopause.

▼ Oats can be useful in incidents of drug withdrawal.

▼ Oats may ease heart palpitations.

▼ Diluted infusions of oats may be carefully given to children for colic and stomach problems.

▼ Commercial preparations of oat straw can be added to warm baths to relieve skin conditions.

Preparation and Dosage

Oat products are most commonly available in commercial form as capsules, extracts, infusions, and tinctures.

Capsules: Up to 10 #0 capsules three times daily.

Extract: 1 teaspoon up to three times daily.

Infusion: Up to 3 cups daily.

Tincture: 1 teaspoon up to three times daily.

General Precautions

Oats are a very safe herb, but normal precautions should be taken with any remedy.

▲

PAPAYA (*Carica papaya*)

Papaya, also known as papaw and melon tree, is nature's perfect digestive aid. Papaya contains a number of important digestive enzymes. Papain, similar to the human enzyme pepsin, helps the body break down meat and dairy products. Another enzyme in papaya, chymopapain, has been approved by the United States Food and Drug Administration to help shrink herniated or slipped disks.

You can simply begin your meal with a slice of delicious ripe papaya to ensure that you will digest the meal well. You can also chew on a tasty tablet. Either way, papaya is a safe and natural alternative to the antacids that many people often find themselves popping all day. Over time, overuse of antacids can backfire, because in response your stomach may eventually begin to produce even more acid. Papaya does not have this effect on your body.

Parts Used: Fruit, latex (milky fluid from mature but not yet ripe papayas), leaves, and seeds.

Primary Functions

▼ Papaya is an excellent digestive aid. Use it to relieve an upset stomach.

Other Benefits

▼ Papaya may help prevent ulcers.
▼ Papaya may help get rid of intestinal parasites.

Preparation and Dosage

Papaya products are most commonly available in commercial form as fresh fruit and juice, capsules, and infusions.

Fresh Fruit and Juice: Enjoy fresh papaya in season.

Capsules: 1 capsule up to three times daily.

Infusion: 1 cup during or after a meal, especially when the food you eat is high in protein.

General Precautions

Papaya is generally a safe herb, but normal precautions should be taken with any remedy. Since medicinal amounts of papaya have a reputation for bringing on delayed periods, avoid papaya infusions and tablets if you are or suspect you may be pregnant. Don't worry about eating moderate amounts of ripe papaya fruit. There have been occasional reports of allergic reactions, such as asthma.

PARSLEY (*Petroselinum sativum*)

Parsley contains two important chemicals, apiole and myristicin, that have significant diuretic and mild laxative qualities. Parsley can help you eliminate bloating and excess water weight. It can ease the pain of flatulence (gas) and colic, and has a reputation for bringing on delayed or suppressed menstruation. Parsley is also rich in vitamins A and C.

Parts Used: Root, leaves, and seeds.

Primary Functions

▼ Parsley is an effective diuretic for eliminating excess water weight.

▼ Parsley freshens your breath.

▼ Parsley may relieve gas and colic.

Other Benefits

▼ Parsley may stimulate menstruation.

▼ Parsley may be taken to relieve the bloating that many women experience due to PMS.

▼ In one study, parsley was shown to have antihistamine qualities, which may make it useful in relieving allergy symptoms.

Preparation and Dosage

Parsley products are most commonly available in commercial form as fresh sprigs, infusions, and tinctures.

Fresh Sprigs: Enjoy fresh parsley: it freshens your breath and is packed with vitamins A and C.

Infusion: Up to 3 cups daily.

Tincture: 1/2 to 1 teaspoon up to three times daily.

General Precautions

Parsley is generally a safe herb, but normal precautions should be taken with any remedy. Large amounts of parsley (as in infusions and tinctures) should not be used during pregnancy, since this may stimulate the womb. Incorporating normal amounts of parsley into your diet is no problem.

▲

PAU D'ARCO (*Tabebuia heptaphylla*)

Pau d'arco, also known as lapacho, is the bark of a tree native to Brazil. It has proven to be one of nature's best fungus fighters, an effective treatment for annoying ailments such as athlete's foot and vaginal yeast infections. Pau d'arco is also reputed to lower blood sugar levels and aid the digestive process.

In addition, pau d'arco contains the active constituent laprachol, which investigation has shown may have anti-cancer potential. While the use of laprachol as a cancer fighter is still in the research stage, other studies have shown that laprachol may help kill parasites.

Parts Used: Bark (especially the inner bark).

Primary Functions

▼ Pau d'arco is a good remedy for fungal infections.

▼ Pau d'arco may be an adjunct to regular treatment of adult-onset diabetes, since it said to lower blood sugar. Since diabetes is a serious disease, consult with your physician before incorporating any extras into your medical regimen.

Other Benefits

▼ Exciting new studies have shown that pau d'arco may prove to be a valuable anticarcinogen.

▼ Pau d'arco is good for your digestion.

▼ Pau d'arco may also be a remedy for parasitic infections.

Preparation and Dosage

Pau d'arco products are most commonly available in commercial form as capsules, decoctions, extracts, and tinctures.

Capsules: 1 capsule up to three times daily.

Decoction: 1 cup up to three times daily.

Extract: Mix 25 to 40 drops in water or juice up to three times daily.

Tincture: 1 teaspoon up to three times daily.

General Precautions

Pau d'arco is a very safe herb, but normal precautions should be taken with any remedy.

▲

PEPPERMINT (*Mentha piperita*)

Peppermint is a traditional home remedy for colds, flu, and digestive upsets. Peppermint relieves fever and chills. Because it contains a volatile oil that relaxes the stomach, peppermint is used for a wide range of digestive problems, such as flatulence (gas), nausea, vomiting, heartburn, and diarrhea. Some use peppermint as a tonic to relieve tension and stress. A peppermint infusion is also a healthy and tasty alternative to ordinary tea and coffee.

Parts Used: Leaves.

Primary Functions

▼ Peppermint is most useful in the treatment of fevers, colds, and flu.

▼ Peppermint can relieve gas and a variety of other digestive disturbances, including stomachaches, colic, nausea, vomiting, heartburn, and diarrhea.

Other Benefits

▼ Peppermint may be taken as a tonic to relieve stress, anxiety, and tension.

▼ If you suffer from insomnia, 1 cup of peppermint tea may help you get a good night's sleep.

▼ A few drops of peppermint in hot water can open your sinuses or provide a quick facial.

Preparation and Dosage

Peppermint products are most commonly available in commercial form as infusions and oils.

Infusion: Drink as often as desired.

Oil: Use 10 drops of peppermint oil in proportion to 2 quarts of hot water.

General Precautions

Peppermint is a very safe herb, but normal precautions should be taken with any remedy.

▲

PLANTAIN (*Plantago major*)

Plantain is valued for its healing qualities when used internally and externally. Internally, plantain is a soothing remedy for coughs and bronchitis. Plantain also contains an active constituent called aucubin, which makes it valuable in the treatment of urinary-tract infections. Its astringent qualities can help you clear up a bout with diarrhea. Externally, plantain ointment may be used to treat hemorrhoids, wounds, bites, and stings.

Parts Used: Leaves.

Primary Functions

▼ Plantain is useful in the treatment of coughs and bronchitis.

▼ Plantain is valuable in the treatment of urinary-tract infections.

Other Benefits

▼ Plantain is a mild expectorant.

▼ Plantain may relieve diarrhea.

▼ Plantain ointment may help heal hemorrhoids, wounds, bites, and stings.

Preparation and Dosage

Plantain products are most commonly available in commercial form as infusions, tinctures, and ointments.

Infusion: 1 cup up to three times daily.

Tincture: 1 teaspoon up to three times daily.

Ointment: Apply locally as needed.

General Precautions

Plantain is a very safe herb, but normal precautions should be taken with any remedy.

▲

PSYLLIUM (*Plantago psyllium*)

Psyllium, which is also known as fleaseed or plantago, is one of nature's safest and gentlest laxatives. In fact, psyllium is the major ingredient in some of the most popular commercial laxatives, including Fiberall, Hydrocil, Metamucil, Pro-Lax, and N-Lax.

Psyllium is a bulking laxative, useful in most cases of irritable or sluggish digestion. Psyllium seeds are coated with a substance called mucilage, which absorbs water. You should always drink a lot of water when taking psyllium seeds: they work by absorbing water and thus increasing the bulk, or size, of stools in the bowel. Larger stools in turn press on the colon, stimulating the muscles, which move the stools along and result in a bowel movement.

Parts Used: Seeds.

Primary Functions

▼ Psyllium is a safe and gentle natural laxative.

Other Benefits

▼ Recent studies have also shown that psyllium, which is rich in soluble fiber, has the capacity to reduce blood cholesterol levels.

Preparation and Dosage

Psyllium products are most commonly available in commercial form as seeds, capsules, and infusions. Remember to drink plenty of water with all psyllium products.

Seeds: 1 teaspoon of crushed seeds or powder up to three times daily with meals. You may also use the husks.

Capsules: 6 to 8 #0 capsules up to three times daily.

Infusions: 2 to 4 teaspoons after each meal.

General Precautions

Psyllium is generally a safe herb, but you must remember how psyllium seeds work—that is, by absorbing water. The seeds soak up water and add bulk to your stools. If you do not take water with psyllium, you may wind up increasing the constipation you are seeking to get rid of.

Pregnant women should avoid all laxatives. A qualified professional should be consulted before psyllium is taken by nursing women or administered to children.

RASPBERRY (*Rubus idaeus*)

Raspberry leaves are a natural tonic that can strengthen and tone the womb. They are one of the few herbs that are used during pregnancy, and are especially useful in assisting contractions during labor. Of course, no remedy should be taken during pregnancy without first consulting a qualified professional.

Ancient Greek, Chinese, and Ayurvedic herbalists recommended raspberry as a treatment for wounds and diarrhea. Today it is still used for diarrhea and mouth problems such as bleeding gums. Gargling with raspberry may relieve the pain of a sore throat.

Parts Used: Leaves.

Primary Functions

▼ Raspberry is a natural uterine tonic. It is a helpful addition to most women's remedies, as in fertility formulas. Under the guidance of a qualified professional, raspberry may be used during the last trimester of pregnancy.

Other Benefits

▼ Raspberry may be used to treat diarrhea.

▼ Raspberry may be helpful in the relief of mouth problems and sore throats.

▼ A recent study has shown that raspberry has the capacity to reduce blood sugar.

Preparation and Dosage

Raspberry products are most commonly available in commercial form as infusions and tinctures.

Infusion: 1 cup up to three times daily.
Tincture: 1 teaspoon up to three times daily.

General Precautions

Raspberry is a very safe herb, but normal precautions should be taken with any remedy.

▲

RED CLOVER (*Trifolium pratense*)

Red clover—also known as cow clover, purple clover, and trifolium—has long had a great reputation as an immune enhancer with possible anticancer qualities. Researchers at the National Cancer Institute have recently discovered that red clover does indeed have certain antitumor properties. Red clover contains antitumor compounds such as genistein and the antioxidant tocopherol, which is a form of vitamin E that has prevented breast tumors in animal studies. Many herbalists recommend red clover as a valuable supplement to the conventional medical treatment of HIV/AIDS and cancer (especially of the breast and ovaries).

Red clover has a long history of herbal use, dating back to the ancient Greeks and Romans. Today this versatile herb is still used to treat a wide host of symptoms and ailments. It is considered an especially effective remedy for skin problems such as eczema, especially in children. The expectorant qualities of red clover make this herb helpful as a treatment for whooping cough, other types of coughs, and bronchitis.

Parts Used: Flower heads.

Primary Functions

▼ Red clover has immune-enhancing properties that may make it a helpful supplemental treatment for HIV/ AIDS.

▼ Red clover may be useful in preventing or treating certain types of cancer. It may act as a valuable adjunct to traditional medical treatment of cancer.

▼ Red clover is also a remedy for a variety of skin ailments, such as eczema and psoriasis. It is thought to be especially helpful for children.

Other Benefits

▼ Red clover has expectorant properties that make it useful in treating coughs (especially whooping cough) and bronchitis.

▼ Red clover may act as a digestive aid.

▼ Large doses of red clover may act in a manner similar to estrogen. Because of this, it may help alleviate some of the symptoms of menopause.

Preparation and Dosage

Red clover products are most commonly available in commercial form as infusions and tinctures.

Infusion: 1 cup up to three times daily.

Tincture: ½ to 1½ teaspoons up to three times daily.

General Precautions

Red clover is a very safe and potentially extremely beneficial herb. Simply observe normal precautions.

ROSEMARY (*Rosmarinus officinalis*)

Rosemary has been used since ancient times, when Greek students wore rosemary necklaces to improve their memories. While this particular quality of rosemary remains unproven, we do use rosemary today to stimulate the nervous system. Rosemary also has a tonic effect upon the circulatory and digestive systems. It relaxes the muscles of the digestive tract—which, along with its preservative qualities, may account for its long culinary use. Rosemary is recommended for a variety of ailments, ranging from depression to muscle aches and pains.

Parts Used: Leaves.

Primary Functions

▼ Rosemary acts as a stimulant to the circulatory, digestive, and nervous systems.

Other Benefits

▼ Rosemary may be taken internally to relieve headache pain.

▼ Rosemary contains antioxidant chemicals; cooking with rosemary may help prevent food poisoning.

▼ The oil of rosemary can be rubbed on your temples to ease the pain of headaches, especially migraines.

▼ Try adding oil of rosemary to your bath for a little extra relaxation.

▼ Rosemary can soothe sore muscles.

Preparation and Dosage

Rosemary products are most commonly available in

commercial form as infusions, tinctures, and oils. Keep in mind that rosemary oil is for external use only.

Infusion: 1 cup up to three times daily.

Tincture: ¼ to ½ teaspoon up to three times daily.

Oil: Rub on the temples to provide relief from headaches. Toss a little in your bath for relaxation.

General Precautions

The oil of rosemary should only be used externally. Since rosemary has a traditional (although unproven) reputation of bringing on delayed menstrual periods, it's better to err on the side of safety: feel free to use rosemary in your cooking, but avoid taking medicinal amounts of rosemary if you are or suspect you may be pregnant. Nursing women should take rosemary only after conferring with a qualified professional.

▲

ST. JOHN'S WORT (*Hypericum perforatum*)

St. John's wort is a highly valued herb that has been used in healing for more than two thousand years. Because it contains both immune-enhancing and antiviral components, this herb has been heartily welcomed by many AIDS researchers. St. John's wort has significant concentrations of immune-modulating flavonoids, and also contains hypericin, a substance that is both antiviral and antidepressive.

St. John's wort holds a wealth of wonderful healing possibilities. In addition to its exciting potential as a treatment for HIV/AIDS, St. John's wort may act as a natural antidepressant, and provides valuable relief to those suffering from anxiety, tension, and stress. Tension headaches may also respond well to treatment with St. John's wort.

St. John's wort is a common herbal recommendation for menstrual cramps and the symptoms of menopause. And, because St. John's wort also has antiviral properties, it may act as an effective remedy for attacks of herpes simplex, which are often brought on by stress. Externally, this extraordinarily versatile herb is used in the **healing** of bruises, minor burns (such as sunburn), psoriasis, varicose veins, and wounds.

Parts Used: Flowers and leaves.

Primary Functions

▼ St. John's wort may be used in the treatment of depression, as well as in the relief of everyday stress.

▼ St. John's wort often relieves menstrual cramps and some of the symptoms of menopause, such as anxiety and irritability.

▼ St. John's wort is a valuable healing remedy for external problems, such as bruises, minor burns, psoriasis, varicose veins, and wounds.

Other Benefits

▼ Scientists are currently studying the impact that St. John's wort may have on HIV/AIDS. While no definitive results have been established, early anecdotal reports seem promising.

▼ St. John's wort may be an effective remedy for herpes simplex.

▼ St. John's wort may relieve the pain of tension headaches.

▼ St. John's wort is sometimes used in the treatment of sciatica and rheumatic pain.

Preparation and Dosage

St. John's wort products are most commonly available in commercial form as infusions, tinctures, lotions, and oils.

Infusion: 1 cup up to three times daily.

Tincture: 1/4 to 1 teaspoon up to three times daily.

Lotion: Apply locally as needed to bruises, minor burns, psoriasis, varicose veins, and wounds.

Oil: Apply locally to sunburn.

Special Precautions

Large doses of St. John's wort may make fair-skinned individuals especially sensitive to the sun. If you fall into this category, stay out of the sun to avoid getting a sunburn while taking St. John's wort. Otherwise, this is a very safe herb.

▲

SAW PALMETTO (*Serenoa serrulata*)

Saw palmetto can be a boost to the male reproductive system. It may increase a man's fertility, ease cases of benign prostate enlargement, and is even reputed to act as an aphrodisiac.

Saw palmetto has other herbal applications as well.

The expectorant properties of saw palmetto can help ease all kinds of congestion. It may be useful in various respiratory conditions, such as asthma, bronchitis, colds, and coughs.

Parts Used: Berries.

Primary Functions

▼ Saw palmetto may increase male fertility.

▼ Saw palmetto may help in the treatment of benign prostate enlargement.

Other Benefits

▼ Saw palmetto is said to be an aphrodisiac for men.

▼ The expectorant qualities of saw palmetto may make it valuable in the treatment of asthma, bronchitis, colds, and coughs.

Preparation and Dosage

Saw palmetto products are most commonly available in commercial form as capsules, infusions, extracts, and tinctures.

Capsules: 2 to 4 #0 capsules up to three times daily.

Infusion: 1 cup up to three times daily.

Extract: Mix 30 to 60 drops in water or juice, taken daily.

Tincture: 1 teaspoon up to three times daily.

General Precautions

Saw palmetto is generally a safe and beneficial herb, but men who suffer from prostate conditions should take care to consult a qualified professional. Normal precautions should of course be taken with any herbal remedy.

▲

SLIPPERY ELM (*Ulmus rubra*)

Slippery elm, which is also known as Indian elm or red elm, contains a gentle and nutritive substance called mucilage, which can help ease digestive problems such as colitis, diarrhea, duodenal ulcers, and gastritis. Its soothing qualities also make slippery elm a valuable treatment for coughs, colds, and sore throats. Externally, a slippery elm poultice may be applied to abscesses, boils, burns, and wounds.

Parts Used: Bark.

Primary Functions
▼ Slippery elm is often used in the treatment of inflamed digestive conditions, such as colitis, diarrhea, duodenal ulcers, enteritis, and gastritis.

Other Benefits
▼ Slippery elm may soothe coughs, colds, and sore throats.
▼ Slippery elm can be made into a poultice to treat external problems such as abscesses, boils, minor burns, and wounds.

Preparation and Dosage

Slippery elm products are most commonly available in commercial form as capsules, decoctions, tinctures, and poultices.

Capsules: Take as directed.

Decoction: 1 cup up to three times daily.

Tincture: 1 teaspoon up to three times daily.

Poultice: Make a paste of powdered bark and water; apply locally as needed.

General Precautions

Slippery elm is a very safe herb, but normal precautions should of course be taken with any herbal remedy.

▲

THYME (*Thymus vulgaris*)

Thyme has a long herbal history as an external antiseptic and, when used internally, as both a respiratory and digestive aid. The aromatic oil of thyme contains two active constituents—thymol and carvacrol—that account for these qualities. In fact, thymol was a major antiseptic used by wounded soldiers through World War I, after which it was replaced by more effective manufactured drugs.

Today thyme is still an appropriate herbal remedy for minor cuts and scrapes. Its antiseptic qualities make it a natural addition to a number of commercial products, such as Listerine. Thyme is an expectorant, which makes it useful in the treatment of coughs and colds; in fact, thyme enjoys great popularity in respiratory remedies used in Germany today. Thyme is also soothing and relaxing to the digestive tract, and is safe and gentle enough to treat diarrhea in children.

Parts Used: Leaves and flowers.

Primary Functions

▼ Thyme may alleviate indigestion.

▼ Thyme is gentle enough to help relieve children's diarrhea.

▼ Thyme is a cough remedy.

▼ Thyme lotion is a natural anesthetic for minor wounds.

Other Benefits

▼ Thyme may be used for a variety of other respiratory problems, such as asthma, bronchitis, emphysema, and whooping cough.

▼ Thyme may be a helpful remedy for cases of laryngitis, tonsillitis, and general sore throats.

▼ Thyme may relieve menstrual cramps.

Preparation and Dosage

Thyme products are most commonly available in commercial form as infusions, tinctures, and lotions. Do not use the oil that is sometimes extracted from thyme; it has toxic effects when taken internally.

Infusion: 1 cup up to three times daily.

Tincture: ½ to 1 teaspoon up to three times daily.

Lotion: Apply locally as needed to disinfect minor cuts and scrapes.

General Precautions

While small amounts of thyme are said to relieve menstrual cramps, large amounts may act as uterine stimulants. Culinary amounts of thyme are fine to use in your cooking while pregnant; but just to be on the safe side, avoid taking infusions and tinctures of thyme if you are or suspect you may be pregnant.

Otherwise, thyme is a safe and helpful herb. Diluted amounts of thyme are even considered gentle enough to treat diarrhea in children. When in doubt, of course, consult a qualified professional.

Normal precautions apply to all remedies.

UVA-URSI (*Arctostaphylos uva-ursi*)

Uva-ursi, which is also commonly known as bearberry, is a natural tonic for your urinary system. It soothes and strengthens urinary membranes and may help relieve infections such as cystitis. Uva-ursi is specifically effective in cases of highly acidic urine.

Active constituents in uva-ursi account for these valuable healing abilities. Arbutin, ursolic acid, and allantoin are among the many chemicals that contribute to the overall antiseptic and diuretic effect of this herb.

Parts Used: Leaves.

Primary Functions

▼ Uva-ursi nurtures and strengthens the urinary system. It may help in the treatment of certain urinary-tract infections.

Other Benefits

▼ Because of its diuretic qualities, uva-ursi may relieve premenstrual bloating.

▼ Diuretics are also taken as part of the treatment of serious medical problems, such as high blood pressure and congestive heart failure. Speak to your physician about incorporating natural diuretics into your regular medical regimen.

Preparation and Dosage

Uva-ursi products are most commonly available in commercial form as infusions and tinctures.

Infusion: 1 cup up to three times daily.

Tincture: ¼ to 1 teaspoon up to three times daily.

Special Precautions

Because uva-ursi is a diuretic—that is, it promotes urine production—it should not be used by pregnant or nursing women.

Uva-ursi is similar to juniper, in that it should never be used if the kidneys are involved. For example, do not use uva-ursi if you are experiencing lower-back pain, which can be a symptom of kidney disease. Consult a professional in these cases.

One side effect of uva-ursi is that it may turn your urine dark green. This is a natural side effect, and—odd as it may seem to you at first—you should not become alarmed by it. Side effects that you *should* watch out for and report to your herbalist or herbally oriented physician are nausea and ringing in the ears. A qualified professional should also be informed if you have a prior medical condition or are taking other medications.

If the dosage on the label of an uva-ursi remedy is stated in terms of a range, begin use with the lowest dosage. Because diuretics deplete your potassium level, eat a lot of potassium-packed bananas or take a potassium supplement along with uva-ursi. Parents should consult with their pediatrician before administering uva-ursi to children.

▲

VALERIAN (*Valeriana officinalis*)

Although chemically unrelated to the tranquilizer Valium, valerian has been nicknamed "the Valium of the nineteenth century." In fact, it is said that Valium was named for valerian. Valerian is a safe and natural alternative to sedative drugs such as Valium, and it is used worldwide to relieve nervous tension and stress. For centuries, herbalists have used valerian to treat panic attacks. And, unlike prescription drugs, valerian has the great advantage of not being addictive.

Primary Functions
▼ Valerian can help relieve tension and stress.
▼ Valerian is often used to treat insomnia.
▼ Valerian may ease menstrual cramps and PMS.

Other Benefits

▼ Valerian can relieve gas and intestinal cramps.

▼ Valerian may be useful in treating low fevers and colds.

Preparation and Dosage

Valerian products are most commonly available in commercial form as infusions, tinctures, and capsules.

Infusion: 1 cup before bedtime.

Tincture: 1 teaspoon up to three times daily.

Capsules: As directed.

Special Precautions

Valerian is generally a safe herb, but since it may create a sleepy effect it is best not to drive while taking valerian. It is especially important to follow the recommended dosages on the labels of valerian products. An overdosage of valerian could result in a dangerous weakening of the heartbeat. If you should experience an upset stomach while taking valerian, try taking your recommended dosage at mealtime.

▲

VERVAIN (*Verbena officinalis*)

Vervain—which is also known as herb-of-the-cross, simpler's joy, and verbena—has been used since ancient times for a wide assortment of symptoms and ailments. Hippocrates recommended vervain for the treatment of fever and plague. Native Americans also used vervain to relieve fever and to alleviate stomach problems.

Today vervain is used to treat fevers, and some herbalists recommend vervain to relieve mild pain and reduce inflammation. Vervain also has a tranquilizing effect and can be used to ease everyday tension and stress.

Parts Used: Flowers and leaves.

Primary Functions
- ▼ Vervain may relieve tension and stress.
- ▼ Vervain may relieve fevers.

Other Benefits
- ▼ Because it has some aspirinlike effects, vervain may be used in the treatment of simple headaches, toothaches, and wounds.
- ▼ Vervain may reduce inflammations.
- ▼ Vervain may provide mild pain relief.

Preparation and Dosage
Vervain products are most commonly available in commercial form as infusions and tinctures.

Infusion: 1 cup before bedtime.

Tincture: 1 teaspoon up to three times daily.

General Precautions
Vervain is a very safe herb, but normal precautions should be taken with any herbal remedy.

VITEX *See agnus-castus*

WHITE WILLOW (*Salix alba*)

White willow, also known as salicin willow, is the original herbal aspirin. Like meadowsweet, white willow contains an aspirinlike chemical called salicin. Salicin is the precursor of aspirin: it relieves pain, reduces fever, and has anti-inflammatory qualities. White willow is especially beneficial because it does not cause the stomach upset that many people experience when they take aspirin. In fact, one of the constituents in white willow—tannin—is a digestive aid.

Today many people use white willow as a mild alternative to aspirin. It contains more salicylates than meadowsweet, meaning that it is an even more powerful healing agent. Like aspirin, white willow reduces fever, pain, and inflammation. Women take white willow to relieve menstrual cramps; the salicylate in white willow acts to suppress prostaglandins, which are a causal factor in menstrual cramps.

Parts Used: Bark.

Primary Functions
▼ White willow is a good remedy for fevers.
▼ White willow is used to relieve headaches and other pains.
▼ White willow may soothe inflammatory conditions such as arthritis and rheumatism.

206

Other Benefits

▼ Some research suggests that white willow may play a role in lowering blood sugar.

▼ White willow may ease menstrual cramps.

Preparation and Dosage

White willow products are most commonly available in commercial form as capsules, decoctions, and tinctures.

Capsules: Follow the directions on the label. Usually these will mirror those of aspirin: 2 capsules every three to four hours.

Decoction: Up to 3 cups daily.

Tincture: 1 teaspoon up to three times daily.

Special Precautions

To be on the safe side, pregnant women should not take white willow, since studies have shown that aspirin, which is chemically similar to white willow, may increase your risk of birth defects.

White willow is not an appropriate remedy for children under two, or for children under sixteen who are suffering from a cold, fever, flu, or chicken pox. This is because white willow closely resembles aspirin, which has been linked with Reye Syndrome, a potentially fatal condition associated with children's fevers. While there has been no direct evidence linking white willow with Reye Syndrome, it is better to err on the side of caution: avoid giving this herb to feverish children.

WILD CHERRY BARK (*Prunus serotina*)

Wild cherry bark is the classic remedy for coughs. It was a favorite cure of nineteenth-century physicians, and it is still used to flavor children's cold and cough medications. Wild cherry bark is a good treatment for coughs, colds, bronchitis, and asthma. Wild cherry loosens phlegm and has a mild sedative quality, and is also thought to be helpful in a variety of digestive disorders.

Parts Used: Bark.

Primary Functions
▼ Wild cherry bark is an excellent remedy for coughs, colds, bronchitis, and asthma.

Other Benefits
▼ Wild cherry bark may be helpful in the treatment of colitis, diarrhea, gastritis, and ulcers.

▼ Wild cherry bark has a mild sedative effect.

Preparation and Dosage
Wild cherry bark products are most commonly available in commercial form as infusions and tinctures.

Infusion: 1 cup up to three times daily.

Tincture: $1/4$ to $1/2$ teaspoon up to three times daily.

· Special Precautions
Pregnant women should not take wild cherry bark; it has been associated with birth defects in animal studies.

It is important to pay close attention to dosages of wild cherry bark. This herb contains large amounts of hydrocyanic acid, which in large quantities can be toxic. Carefully follow the dosage schedule of wild cherry bark, beginning use with the lowest recommended dosage.

Nursing women should take wild cherry bark only after conferring with their obstetrician or midwife. Parents should consult with their pediatrician before administering wild cherry bark to children.

▲

WILD INDIGO (*Baptisia tinctoria*)

Wild indigo, also known as horsefly weed, is a natural infection fighter. This herb contains alkaloids and flavonoids that make it especially effective in treating infections of the ear, nose, throat, and lymph glands. Wild indigo also helps reduce fevers. A mouthwash made of wild indigo may help soothe and heal mouth ulcers and gingivitis. Wild indigo ointment can relieve sore nipples.

Parts Used: Root.

Primary Functions
▼ Wild indigo is especially effective in treating infections of the ear, nose, throat, and lymph glands. Try it when you are suffering from laryngitis or tonsillitis.

Other Benefits
▼ Wild indigo can help reduce fevers.
▼ A mouthwash of wild indigo may heal mouth ulcers and gingivitis.
▼ Try wild indigo ointment to ease sore nipples.

Preparation and Dosage

Wild indigo products are most commonly available in commercial form as decoctions, tinctures, and mouthwashs.

Decoction: 1 cup up to three times daily.

Tincture: 1 teaspoon up to three times daily.

Mouthwash: Gargle as needed.

General Precautions

Wild indigo is a very safe herb, but normal precautions should be taken with any herbal remedy.

▲

WITCH HAZEL (*Hamamelis virginiana*)

You can find a bottle of commercial witch hazel tucked in the back of most American medicine cabinets today. Witch hazel is also an ingredient in a number of other commercial remedies, including Tucks and Preparation H— both used for the treatment of hemorrhoids. In addition, this preparation is a good local remedy for bruises, varicose veins, and wounds.

There is a difference between the distilled witch hazel widely sold in drugstores and the more potent variety found in herb shops and health food stores. The distilled version lacks the astringent tannins that have a more powerful binding action on tissues and help stop bleeding. While some herbalists prepare infusions of witch hazel that can be taken internally, if you are on your own it is best to stick to the external application of witch hazel liquid or ointment.

Parts Used: Bark and leaves.

Primary Functions

▼ Witch hazel may be an effective external remedy for bruises, hemorrhoids, varicose veins, and wounds.

Preparation and Dosage

Witch hazel products are most commonly available in commercial form as liquids and ointments.

Liquid and Ointment: Apply locally as needed.

General Precautions

Witch hazel is intended for external use. If witch hazel causes skin irritations, stop using or dilute. Do not attempt to take witch hazel internally, except under the specific guidance of a qualified herbalist.

▲

WOOD BETONY (*Betonica officinalis*)

Wood betony, which is also known as betony, is one of the classic herbal headache remedies. It is particularly effective in relieving nervous headaches—that is, headaches caused by stress and anxiety. Wood betony nurtures the nervous system and also has a sedative action. This herb has helped many people through a nervous convalescence.

Parts Used: Aboveground parts.

Primary Functions

▼ Wood betony relieves headaches, especially those due to stress and nervous tension.

Other Benefits

▼ Wood betony may relieve general stress and anxiety.

▼ Wood betony may act as a stimulant to your digestive system.

Preparation and Dosage

Wood betony products are most commonly available in commercial form as infusions and tinctures.

Infusion: 1 cup up to three times daily.

Tincture: 1 teaspoon up to three times daily.

General Precautions

Wood betony is a very safe herb, but normal precautions should be taken with any herbal remedy.

▲

YARROW (*Achillea millefolium*)

It is said that yarrow was used by Achilles during the Trojan War to treat soldiers' wounds. And it turns out that Achilles had the right idea! Yarrow contains a number of active constituents—including azulene, camphor, eugenol, rutin, salicylic acid, and tannins—that relieve pain and speed the healing of wounds.

Yarrow—also known as bloodwort, herbe militaire,

nosebleed, soldier's woundwort, staunchgrass, and thousand seal—has a wide variety of other healing qualities. Herbalists recommend yarrow for the treatment of bruises, colds, fevers, hypertension, and sore throats. Another chemical in yarrow—thujone—has a mild sedative effect.

Parts Used: Flowers, leaves, and stems.

Primary Functions

▼ Yarrow is an excellent treatment for wounds, both internally and externally.

▼ Yarrow is used to treat colds and sore throats.

▼ Yarrow is traditionally used to break fevers.

Other Benefits

▼ Yarrow is a mild digestive aid.

▼ Yarrow may relieve menstrual cramps.

▼ Yarrow may have a moderate sedative effect.

▼ Yarrow can be taken internally if you bruise easily.

▼ Yarrow may be taken in cases of hypertension.

Preparation and Dosage

Yarrow products are most commonly available in commercial form as infusions, tinctures, and salves.

Infusion: 1 cup up to three times daily.

Tincture: 1 teaspoon up to three times daily.

Salve: Apply locally as needed.

General Precautions

Yarrow is a very safe herb. A side effect of taking yarrow may be darkened urine; this is normal, and you should not become alarmed about it. Recommended doses of yarrow are safe—but very large amounts of its constituent thujone can be poisonous.

▲

YELLOW DOCK (*Rumex crispus*)

Yellow dock is a versatile herb used in a wide variety of conditions. Because it stimulates the flow of bile, it is an excellent liver and gallbladder tonic. Yellow dock contains active constituents called anthraquinones that have an active effect on the bowel and may ease cases of constipation. Yellow dock is also helpful in conditions ranging from acne to psoriasis to AIDS.

Parts Used: Root.

Primary Functions

▼ Yellow dock is an excellent liver and gallbladder tonic.

▼ Yellow dock may be helpful in cases of constipation.

▼ Yellow dock is used to relieve acne, psoriasis, and other irritated skin conditions.

Other Benefits

▼ Yellow dock may help in the treatment of hemorrhoids and varicose veins.

▼ Yellow dock is often used as a valuable herbal supplement to conventional medical treatment of serious conditions such as HIV/AIDS and cancer.

▼ Yellow dock is high in iron, so it may be useful in cases of anemia.

▼ Yellow dock may help in the care of jaundice.

Preparation and Dosage

Yellow dock products are most commonly available in commercial form as decoctions and tinctures.

Decoction: 1 cup up to three times daily.

Tincture: 1 teaspoon up to three times daily.

General Precautions

Yellow dock is a very safe herb, but normal precautions should be taken with any remedy.

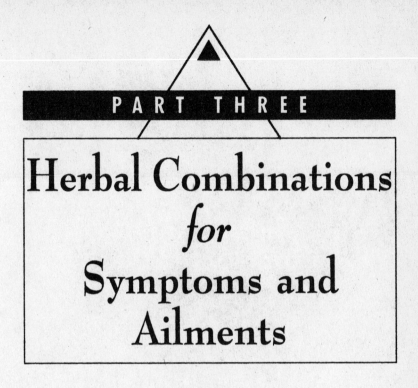

PART THREE

Herbal Combinations *for* Symptoms and Ailments

SYMPTOMS AND AILMENTS:
Which Herbal Remedy Is Right for You?

What's the best herbal remedy for your cold? Which herb do you most frequently reach for when you have a headache? How about when you're nauseated? Is there an herbal remedy to pep you up when you're feeling worn-down?

Each of the herbs we described in Part II has many uses. By looking under "Primary Functions," you can find an herb to treat your headache. Wood betony, for example, is the classic remedy for headaches that are due to tension or stress, while feverfew is a favorite for easing migraine pain. But it is *also* true that many herbs work best synergistically, or in combination with one another. These are some of the remedies that work best.

An Herbal Combination for What Ails You

In Part III you'll find helpful herbal remedies for a wide variety of conditions. Symptoms and ailments are listed in alphabetical order for quick and easy reference. We describe each condition from an herbal point of view and then look at natural actions—especially herbal combinations—that we suggest for the relief of that condition.

Herbal combinations should be used for different periods of time, and how long you use them depends mainly on the severity of the symptom or ailment you are treating. For

219

complete information on the safe use of herbal remedies, see page 18 in Chapter Two.

▼ Minor ailments—such as bad breath, colds, or an occasional inability to get a good night's sleep—usually respond quickly to herbal home care. Remember that your body has a miraculous ability to heal itself. In these cases, herbs are simply helping your body do its work.

▼ Slightly more troublesome symptoms and ailments —such as herpes, psoriasis, sore throats, and urinary-tract infections—are conditions that may respond to herbal treatment. However, if you find that over a period of one to three weeks (depending on the condition) your body is not responding to herbal therapy, seek out the care of a qualified herbalist or medical doctor.

In some chronic cases, such as constipation, we recommend using herbal remedies for intermittent three-month periods. Then take a break and see how you feel. Is it working for you? If the herbs have corrected your condition, you no longer need to take that combination. If you feel worse when you are not taking the remedy, you may wish to return to it. Also, you may want to replace an herb with a different one that has a similar action. When in doubt, consult a qualified herbalist.

▼ Very serious diseases—such as cancer, AIDS, and diabetes, among others—require medical treatment, as may various other potentially serious medical conditions such as asthma and bronchitis. In these cases, herbs can back up drugs, providing a valuable complement to (but not a replacement for) traditional medical care. You should always consult the appropriate medical professional before attempting herbal treatment.

The following is an A to Z guide to symptoms and ailments and our herbal recommendations about how to cope with them. As you read along, keep in mind that your body is an amazing work of art. We have an enormous respect for the human body's ability to heal itself—what we provide are those herbs that can best enable your body to call upon its own natural resources.

▲

ACNE

Acne is a chronic skin disorder caused by inflammation of the sebaceous glands of the skin. Acne can be both painful and embarrassing. It usually begins in puberty, and seems to be linked to fluctuations in the levels of sex hormones. Eliminating fats and sweets from your diet and eating lots of fresh fruit and vegetables may help prevent or eliminate acne. Try to include zinc and vitamins A and D in your diet.

Herbs to treat acne are echinacea and cleavers, which are blood purifiers, and dandelion and yellow dock, which are liver tonics and act as digestive aids. An herbal combination that we recommend for acne includes equal parts of:
- ▼ Cleavers
- ▼ Dandelion
- ▼ Echinacea
- ▼ Yellow dock

Make a decoction by boiling dandelion, echinacea, and yellow dock roots in 1½ pints of water for 10 minutes. Reduce to 1 pint. Add the aboveground parts of cleavers, cover, and steep for another 10 minutes. Use 1 ounce of the total combined herbs recommended, and drink up to three cups daily.

▲

AIDS *(Acquired Immune Deficiency Syndrome)*

Although researchers continue to make progress in AIDS treatments, there is still no cure for AIDS. AIDS is a critical deficiency of the immune system caused by infection with the human immunodeficiency virus (HIV).

Although there is no cure, there are many supportive treatments for the complications of AIDS. A number of remedies are also used to slow the progression of HIV infection.

It's important to remember that the major methods of HIV transmission are sexual contact, sharing needles (as in the case of intravenous drug users), and passage from an infected mother to her fetus. The infection is not spread by casual contact, such as shaking hands or hugging.

AIDS is a life-threatening disease requiring immediate and acute medical care. Many people, whether HIV-positive or already manifesting the symptoms of full-blown AIDS, supplement their standard medical treatment with alternative therapies, including herbal remedies to help boost their immune systems and relieve their symptoms.

Helpful herbal combinations include excellent Chinese immune tonics such as astragalus and ganoderma fungus (which is also called the Reishi mushroom). Isatis is another useful Chinese remedy in the war against AIDS; it is not specifically for the immune system, but has excellent antiviral qualities.

Echinacea and red clover support the immune system, and so they would be appropriate to include in many formulas for HIV/AIDS. Herbalists add other herbs to the combination depending upon what symptoms are present. In this sample combination we have included goldenseal for its valued antiviral and healing respiratory qualities, and licorice, which brings the herbs together in a soothing way. A useful Western combination of herbs consists of equal parts of:

▼ Echinacea
▼ Goldenseal
▼ Licorice
▼ Red clover

Make a decoction by boiling the echinacea, goldenseal, and licorice in 1½ pints of water for 10 minutes. Reduce to 1 pint. Add the aboveground parts of red clover, cover, and steep for an additional 10 minutes. Use 1 ounce of the total combined herbs recommended, and drink 2 to 3 cups of the decoction daily. If you prefer the tincture, take up to 3 teaspoons daily. AIDS is a serious disease. Always seek the advice of a health professional before treating yourself with herbal remedies.

▲

ARTHRITIS

Arthritis is actually an umbrella term for a number of joint diseases, in which one or more of the joints in your body becomes inflamed and painful. It can affect people of all ages, though it is most commonly troubling to older people. It varies in severity from mild aches and pains to severe impairment and joint deformity.

A good natural calcium and magnesium supplement may be helpful. Anti-inflammatory and lymphatic herbs for the treatment of arthritis are cleavers, devil's-claw, and meadowsweet. If there is muscle cramping or tension as well as joint pain, add cramp bark or valerian to the mixture. We recommend an herbal combination including equal parts of:

- ▼ Devil's-claw
- ▼ Cleavers
- ▼ Meadowsweet

Make a decoction by boiling the devil's-claw root in 1½ pints of water for 10 minutes. Reduce to 1 pint. Add the aboveground parts of cleavers and meadowsweet, cover, and steep for another 10 minutes. Use 1 ounce of the total combined herbs recommended, and drink up to 3 cups daily.

▲ ASTHMA

Asthma frequently begins in childhood but is often outgrown. Unfortunately, about one in twenty of us continues to suffer from asthma, with its periodic attacks of breathlessness and wheezing. Some cases of asthma may be triggered by external causes, like pollen or dust; others may simply occur spontaneously. Very severe attacks of asthma can be fatal.

Ephedra, or *ma huang,* is one of the world's oldest herbal remedies for asthma. Ephedra is very potent, so only very small amounts are necessary. You should avoid coffee, tea, colas, and chocolate while taking ephedra; they contain caffeine, and ephedra already has naturally stimulating qualities.

Eliminating dairy products from your diet and taking B-complex vitamins may be helpful in treating asthma. Lobelia and elecampane are beneficial lung tonics, although many people find it hard to stomach the taste of lobelia. If you are one of them, replace the lobelia in the recommended combination with elecampane. Licorice is a soothing relaxant with expectorant qualities. A helpful herbal combination for asthma is:

▼ Ephedra (1 part)
▼ Licorice (2 parts)
▼ Lobelia (1 part)

Make a decoction by boiling the licorice root in 1½ pints of water for 10 minutes. Reduce to 1 pint. Add the aboveground parts of ephedra and lobelia, cover, and steep for another 10 minutes. Use 1 ounce of the total combined herbs recommended, and drink up to 3 cups daily.

▲
ATHLETE'S FOOT

Athlete's foot is a common fungal infection in which the skin between your toes becomes blistered, itchy, and sore. Careful drying of your feet and wearing cotton socks may help.

Topically, a garlic and olive oil salve can ease your discomfort and speed the healing process of athlete's foot. Calendula or myrrh, in ointment or tincture form, can also be rubbed into the affected skin. A helpful herbal combination to clear the blood internally includes equal parts of:

▼ Echinacea
▼ Yellow dock
▼ Cleavers

Make a decoction by boiling the echinacea and yellow dock roots for 10 minutes in 1½ pints of water. Reduce to 1 pint. Add the aboveground parts of cleavers, cover, and steep for an additional 10 minutes. Use 1 ounce of the total combined herbs recommended, and drink up to 3 cups daily.

▲

BAD BREATH

Bad breath is often simply the result of something you ate or drank. Smokers also may have bad breath. Simple herbal remedies for bad breath are chewing on parsley or dill seeds. Sometimes bad breath is the result of poor digestion. A helpful herbal digestive aid consists of equal parts of:

▼ Dandelion
▼ Gentian
▼ Cardamom
▼ Fennel

Make a decoction by boiling the dandelion and gentian roots in 1½ pints of water for 10 minutes. Reduce to 1 pint. Toss in the cardamom and fennel seeds, cover, and steep for another 10 minutes. Use 1 ounce of the total combined herbs recommended, and drink up to 3 cups daily.

▲

BRONCHITIS

Acute or chronic bronchitis is an inflammation of the mucous membranes of your bronchi, airways that connect the windpipe (trachea) and lungs. It is characterized by a persistent cough that often produces considerable amounts of phlegm. Acute bronchitis is usually a bacterial infection that follows a virus (such as colds and flu); chronic bronchitis is most common in smokers and those who live in areas where the air is polluted.

Herbal treatments aim to promote the expectoration of mucus and ease any underlying weakness. Elecampane is particularly good for this. Coltsfoot is helpful in the treatment of dry coughs.

When your cough produces a lot of phlegm, a helpful herbal combination for bronchitis should include equal parts of:

▼ Elecampane
▼ Goldenseal
▼ Licorice

Make a decoction by boiling the three roots in 1½ pints of water for 10 minutes. Reduce to 1 pint. Use 1 ounce of the total combined herbs recommended, and drink up to 3 cups daily.

When bronchitis is accompanied by dry coughs, we recommend treatment with equal parts of:

▼ Licorice
▼ Coltsfoot
▼ Plantain (or mullein)

Make a decoction by boiling the licorice root in 1½ pints of water for 10 minutes. Reduce to 1 pint. Add the aboveground parts of coltsfoot and plantain (or mullein), cover, and steep for another 10 minutes. Use 1 ounce of the total combined herbs recommended, and drink up to 3 cups daily.

▲

BRUISES

Bruises are discolored areas under the skin caused by some sort of injury that causes blood leakage. Severe or unexplained bruises require a professional look. Otherwise, a cloth soaked in ice-cold water can ease the pain and discomfort of a bruise.

Herbal ointments or tinctures made from arnica and/or calendula can be applied topically to bruises. If you bruise easily, vitamin C and rutin are helpful supplements. In addition, a helpful herbal combination to strengthen your blood vessels is:

▼ Horse chestnut
▼ Yarrow

Make an infusion of the aboveground parts of horse

chestnut and yarrow. Cover and steep them in 1 pint of hot water for 10 minutes. Use 1 ounce of the total combined herbs recommended, and drink up to 3 cups daily.

▲

BURNS

Burns in which the skin is broken or blistered require immediate medical attention. First-degree burns—the least serious category—respond to home treatment. These burns cause reddening and affect only the top layer of skin.

Burns should be bathed immediately in cold, running water. There are very effective herbal treatments that you can apply locally as needed on minor burns. Try one or more of these beneficial remedies:

▼ Aloe vera gel
▼ Calendula ointment
▼ St. John's wort oil

▲

CANCER

Cancer is actually a group of diseases in which an unrestrained growth of abnormal cells takes place. Cancer is a critical, life-threatening condition, and requires immediate and aggressive medical intervention. But as in the case of many other serious illnesses, many people choose to complement regular medical care with the care of a qualified herbal practitioner.

Nutritional guidance and vitamin therapy are highly recommended in cancer cases. Herbal treatments of cancer support the immune system and help your body mobilize its natural defenses to get rid of toxins. Echinacea and red clover are immune-enhancing and anticarcinogenic. Yellow dock and dandelion nurture and support the liver, and aid your body in the elimination of toxins. An herbal combination for cancer includes equal parts of:

▼ Dandelion
▼ Echinacea
▼ Yellow dock
▼ Red clover

Make a decoction by boiling the dandelion, echinacea, and yellow dock roots in 1½ pints of water for 10 minutes. Reduce to 1 pint. Add the flower heads of red clover, cover, and steep for another 10 minutes. Use 1 ounce of the total combined herbs recommended, and drink up to 3 cups daily.

If you instead opt for the tincture from a health food store or professional, take up to 3 teaspoons daily. Cancer is a serious disease. Always seek the advice of a health professional before treating yourself with herbal remedies.

▲

CHOLESTEROL, HIGH LEVELS

Cholesterol is a normal part of your body tissues. Too many people, however, suffer from high levels of cholesterol, which clogs the arteries of your heart and can eventually lead to coronary heart disease or stroke.

Exercise and a diet low in fat and high in fresh fruits and vegetables and whole grains can help lower elevated blood cholesterol.

An excellent commercial Chinese remedy to lower cholesterol is Pseudo Ginseng, commonly known in Chinese medicine as Tien Chi. Garlic capsules may also be very helpful. An effective herbal tonic consists of equal parts of:

▼ Ginseng
▼ Hawthorn
▼ Yarrow

Make a decoction by boiling the ginseng root in 1½ pints of water for 10 minutes. Reduce to 1 pint. Add the hawthorn berries and yarrow, cover, and steep for another 10 minutes. Use 1 ounce of the total combined herbs recommended, and drink up to 3 cups daily.

▲

CHRONIC FATIGUE

Chronic fatigue is an immune-deficient or autoimmune disease that can be caused by any number of viruses. Also known as the yuppie flu, chronic fatigue is a sign of exhaustion, of being burned-out on some emotional or physical level. Often people who have chronic fatigue have taken many courses of antibiotics, which over time can deplete the natural immune system.

Chronic fatigue forces you to stop and take a look at

your life, and possibly make some changes. Try to pay more attention to your diet, and engage in stress-reducing techniques such as meditation.

Chronic fatigue responds very well to herbal treatment. Echinacea can boost your immune system, vervain supports the nervous system, and dandelion helps support and detoxify your liver and kidneys. Sometimes damiana, a stimulating tonic, is an effective addition to an herbal remedy for chronic fatigue. A helpful herbal combination for the relief of chronic fatigue should include equal parts of:

▼ Dandelion
▼ Echinacea
▼ Damiana
▼ Vervain

Make a decoction by boiling the dandelion and echinacea roots in 1½ pints of water for 10 minutes. Reduce to 1 pint. Add the aboveground parts of damiana and vervain, cover, and steep for another 10 minutes. Use 1 ounce of the total combined herbs, and drink up to 3 cups daily.

CIRRHOSIS

Cirrhosis is a serious disease of your liver caused by chronic damage to the liver's tissues and cells. Medical intervention is absolutely essential in all cases of cirrhosis. Alcoholism is a major cause of cirrhosis. Since it is the liver's job to remove toxic substances from your blood, abstinence from alcohol, caffeine, and smoking is critical.

In addition to standard medical treatment, herbalism is

rich in remedies that strengthen and detoxify the liver. It is impossible to reverse the damage cirrhosis has already done to your liver—but you *can* prevent further damage. Excellent herbal liver tonics include dandelion and milk thistle. A nutritious and supportive liver tonic includes equal parts of:

▼ Dandelion
▼ Yellow dock
▼ Milk thistle

Make a decoction by boiling the dandelion and yellow dock roots in 1½ pints of water for 10 minutes. Reduce to 1 pint. Then simply toss in the milk thistle seeds, cover, and steep for another 10 minutes. Use 1 ounce of the total combined herbs, and drink up to 3 cups daily.

▲

COLDS

Every year most of us suffer from at least one bout with the stuffy, runny noses, sore throats, and headaches that accompany that classic condition: the common cold.

Colds can be caused by some two hundred viruses. They are passed through droplets in the atmosphere, hand-to-hand contact, and handling contaminated objects. Contrary to popular opinion, colds have nothing to do with avoiding drafty rooms or going out into the cold air with wet hair.

Most colds can be avoided by maintaining our normal resistance to viral infections. But if you do get a cold, good herbal remedies are those that are diaphoretic—that is, they help you work up a good sweat. Raw garlic mixed with honey and ginger tea are two good diaphoretics. And herbs such as elder relieve the feverish conditions associated with ailments of the respiratory system. A helpful internal remedy consists of equal parts of:

▼ Echinacea
▼ Goldenseal
▼ Elder
▼ Peppermint
▼ Yarrow

Make a decoction by boiling the echinacea and goldenseal roots in 1½ pints of water for 10 minutes. Reduce to 1 pint. Add the aboveground portions of elder, peppermint, and yarrow, cover, and steep for an additional 10 minutes. Use 1 ounce of the total combined herbs, and drink up to 3 cups daily.

▲

COLD SORES

Cold sores are small blisters around the mouth caused by a viral infection called herpes simplex. They are a reflection of a slightly damaged immune system. Cold sores tend to occur when you are feeling run-down and your resistance is lowered for some reason. This can happen when you are under a lot of stress, and women often develop cold sores around their menstrual periods.

Try tincture of myrrh or camphor oil applied locally to relieve the pain of cold sores and speed your recovery from them. Zinc and vitamins C and E may also help. Internally,

echinacea is a beneficial herb to support the immune system, and is also a natural antibiotic. Cleavers is a lymphatic
cleanser, while gentian is very cooling and supports the
digestion. A helpful combination of equal parts of these
three herbs can be taken at the first sign of and for the
duration of the cold sores:

▼ Echinacea

▼ Gentian

▼ Cleavers

Make a decoction by boiling the echinacea and gentian
roots in 1½ pints of water for 10 minutes. Reduce to 1 pint.
Add the aboveground portions of cleavers, cover, and steep
for an additional 10 minutes. Use 1 ounce of the total combined herbs, and drink up to 3 cups daily.

COLIC

About one out of every ten babies gets infantile colic.
No one knows exactly what causes colic in young babies,
but it is thought to be due to intestinal spasms. Colicky
babies cry inconsolably, causing themselves—and their
parents—considerable distress.

Drugs are not recommended for very young babies.
Soothing rhythmic activities such as rocking may ease epi-
sodes of colic. Sometimes a drive around the block will do
the trick.

The nursing mother of a colicky baby can also drink a
very mild remedy for colic, which she can pass on to her
baby through her own breast milk. (If you are not nursing,

you might try putting a few drops in baby's formula or milk.) Remember that you should always consult an appropriate medical professional before giving any herbal remedy to infants or children or before taking any herbal remedy if you are nursing. Soothing teas that a mother might drink to relieve her baby's colic are:

▼ Chamomile
▼ Lemon balm

Chamomile and lemon balm are both aboveground parts of plants. Make an infusion of either by covering and steeping them in 1 pint of hot water for 10 minutes. Use 1 ounce per pint of water, and drink up to 3 cups daily.

▲

CONJUNCTIVITIS

Conjunctivitis, also known as pinkeye, is an uncomfortable eye inflammation. Your eye or eyes turn red and bloodshot, and there may be a discharge as well. Herbal eyewashs are a simple and effective remedy for conjunctivitis, and many commercial herbal brands are available. If you want to make your own decoction for external application, try using these herbs for the duration of your condition:

▼ Echinacea (2 parts)
▼ Eyebright (2 parts)
▼ Marigold (1 part)

Make a decoction by boiling the echinacea root in 1½ pints of water for 10 minutes. Reduce to 1 pint. Add the aboveground parts of eyebright and marigold, cover, and steep for an additional 10 minutes. Use as an eyewash up to three times daily.

▲

CONSTIPATION

There are actually two types of constipation. Each has its own source and calls for its own type of treatment.

Atonic Constipation

This type of constipation is due to insufficient fiber in the diet, lack of exercise, and not paying attention to urges to move your bowels. Reversing these habits may take care of the problem.

For relief of atonic constipation, try either psyllium or cascara sagrada, safe and natural laxatives that you can use on a fairly long-term basis. Psyllium is a bulking agent, so if you use it remember to drink plenty of water. Cascara sagrada is a stimulating but very gentle natural laxative. A helpful herbal combination consists of:
- ▼ Cascara sagrada
- ▼ Yellow dock

Make a decoction by boiling the cascara sagrada bark and the yellow dock root in 1½ pints of water for 10 minutes. Reduce to 1 pint. Use 1 ounce of the total combined herbs recommended, and drink up to 3 cups daily. Use this remedy for up to three months at a time; then take a break and start again.

Tense Constipation

Tense constipation is most often found in people with nervous dispositions, and worsens in times of stress. Do not use stimulating laxatives, as they will irritate an already tense condition. A lot of water and fiber in the diet might help move your bowels.

Effective herbal remedies are in the form of capsules; this is because you want the remedy to get through the stomach and reach the intestinal walls. Two types of herbal capsules to take on a short-term basis for this type of constipation are:

▼ Chamomile
▼ Slippery elm

Carefully follow the dosages on the labels of commercial remedies, beginning first with the lowest recommended amount.

Note: If constipation suddenly occurs after a lifetime of normal bowel movements, if there is abdominal pain, or if there is blood in your feces, immediate medical attention is necessary.

COUGHS

The herbal treatment of coughs depends upon the underlying cause and whether they are productive or unproductive coughs. Any cough that persists for more than three days or that is accompanied by other symptoms, such as spitting up blood, requires prompt professional treatment.

Productive Coughs

These are coughs that bring up mucus or phlegm. An herbal remedy for this type of cough is one that will help your body in its effort to eliminate these substances. Elecampane is an especially good expectorant to get the phlegm out when you have a productive cough. A good herbal remedy for this type of cough consists of equal parts of these herbs:

▼ Elecampane
▼ Ginger
▼ Licorice
▼ Lobelia

Make a decoction by boiling the elecampane, ginger, and licorice roots in 1½ pints of water for 10 minutes. Reduce to 1 pint. Add the aboveground portion of lobelia, cover, and steep for an additional 10 minutes. Use 1 ounce of the total combined herbs recommended, and drink up to 3 cups daily for the duration of your cough.

Unproductive Coughs

Unproductive or dry coughs are not associated with mucus or phlegm. Warm and soothing drinks may relieve some of the discomfort brought on by dry coughs. Coltsfoot is the classic herbal remedy for dry coughs. If the cough is very irritating, wild cherry bark, which has a nice relaxing effect, can also be added to the combination. A helpful herbal remedy for dry coughs consists of equal parts of the following herbs:

▼ Licorice
▼ Coltsfoot
▼ Mullein

Make a decoction by boiling the licorice root in 1½ pints of water for 10 minutes. Reduce to 1 pint. Add the aboveground parts of coltsfoot and mullein, cover, and steep for an additional 10 minutes. Use 1 ounce of the total combined herbs recommended, and drink up to 3 cups daily for the duration of your cough.

Note: An equal part of wild cherry bark can be added to this remedy if your cough is persistent and disturbs your sleep. (See page 208 for precautions concerning wild cherry bark.)

▲

DEPRESSION

Herbalists can treat cases of depression with restorative tonics, but it is also very important to identify the underlying cause of your problem. In serious cases of depression it is best to consult a qualified professional. A very stabilizing and supportive herbal combination for depression consists of equal parts of:

▼ Damiana
▼ Oats
▼ St. John's wort
▼ Vervain

Make an infusion of the aboveground parts of all these herbs. Cover and steep them in 1 pint of hot water for 10 minutes. Use 1 ounce of the total combined herbs recommended, and drink up to 3 cups daily.

DIABETES MELLITUS

Diabetes mellitus is a serious disease, and no decisions about herbal treatment should be made without consultation with a qualified practitioner. There are two types of diabetes mellitus.

Type I—juvenile onset—diabetes first appears in children. It is the more severe form of diabetes, requiring regular insulin treatment. Herbal remedies are generally not appropriate for type I diabetics.

The early stages of type II—adult onset—diabetes are more responsive to herbal treatment. In fact, many early cases of type II diabetes are controlled by careful attention to your diet. You might also try taking one or two guar-gum capsules with each meal; guar gum, a dietary fiber, attaches glucose molecules to itself and therefore allows sugar absorption to proceed more slowly. A wonderful herbal tonic for this type of diabetes includes goat's rue and gentian, bitter herbs that help glucose metabolism. A helpful herbal combination consists of equal parts of:

▼ Gentian
▼ Ginseng
▼ Goat's rue

Make a decoction by boiling the gentian and ginseng roots in 1½ pints of water for 10 minutes. Reduce to 1 pint. Add the aboveground parts of goat's rue, cover, and steep for an additional 10 minutes. Use 1 ounce of the total combined herbs recommended, and drink up to 3 cups daily. This remedy is safe enough to take on a fairly long-term basis.

DIARRHEA

Diarrhea is an increase in the fluidity and frequency of your bowel movements. Diarrhea may be either acute or chronic.

Diarrhea is not a disease; it is a symptom of an underlying problem. Because long bouts of diarrhea may deplete your body's supply of fluid and potassium, it's critical to pay careful attention to diarrhea. This is especially important when babies or older people suffer from this condition.

In some instances acute diarrhea is the result of food poisoning and may last from several hours to several days. Cases of food poisoning require immediate medical attention.

Chronic diarrhea can be a sign of a serious underlying disease, such as Crohn's disease or irritable-bowel syndrome. Because the underlying cause must also be treated, serious cases of diarrhea require the attention of a qualified practitioner.

For a mild and transient case of diarrhea, we recommend gentle herbal astringents such as agrimony and meadowsweet, in combination with the very balancing and settling dandelion:

▼ Dandelion
▼ Agrimony
▼ Meadowsweet

Make a decoction by boiling the dandelion root in 1½ pints of water for 10 minutes. Reduce to 1 pint. Add the aboveground parts of agrimony and meadowsweet, cover, and steep for an additional 10 minutes. Use 1 ounce of the total combined herbs recommended, and drink up to 3 cups daily. If this remedy doesn't work over a three-day period, seek professional help.

DIGESTIVE PROBLEMS

Herbalists believe that most digestive problems—such as gas, nausea, vomiting, bloating, or heartburn—can be avoided by careful attention to your lifestyle. Smoking and drinking alcohol irritate the walls of your intestines. Stress can also have a negative impact on your digestive system. Your diet should include plenty of fresh fruits and vegetables, as well as whole grains.

Digestive aids are remedies that help your digestive processes operate more efficiently. Some digestive aids are stimulants, while others are relaxants. When in doubt, consult a qualified herbalist to see which is most appropriate for you.

Digestive Stimulants

If you suffer from sluggish digestion, you probably need a digestive stimulant. We recommend a combination of equal parts of the following herbs:

▼ Dandelion
▼ Gentian
▼ Cardamom
▼ Fenugreek

Make a decoction by boiling the dandelion and gentian roots in 1½ pints of water for 10 minutes. Reduce to 1 pint. Toss in the cardamom and fenugreek seeds, cover, and steep for another 10 minutes. Drink up to 3 cups daily. Take this remedy for up to three months at a time; then take a break and start again.

Digestive Relaxants

If you suffer from nervous overactivity in your digestive system, you probably need a relaxant. A helpful combination consists of equal parts of the following herbs:

▼ Chamomile
▼ Hops
▼ Lemon balm

Make an infusion of the aboveground parts of these herbs. Cover and steep them in 1 pint of hot water for 10 minutes. Use 1 ounce of the total combined herbs recommended, and drink up to 3 cups daily.

▲

DIZZINESS

Dizziness is a feeling of light-headedness and instability. Often dizziness is a mild symptom, caused by a drop in blood pressure. Other forms of dizziness, especially vertigo, are more severe; they are characterized by a sickening sensation of spinning, accompanied by nausea and vomiting. Dizziness is often caused by an imbalance in the middle ear. To relieve dizziness, we recommend taking a combination of equal parts of these herbs:

▼ Ginger
▼ Feverfew

Shave ½ ounce of ginger root and add to ½ ounce of the aboveground parts of feverfew. Cover and steep for 10 minutes. Drink up to 3 cups daily.

EAR PROBLEMS

Herbalists treat irritations of the outer and middle ear with both external and internal remedies. To confirm that the ear drum is undamaged, it is wisest to seek the advice of a qualified professional before using ear drops.

To make an external remedy for ear infections, heat garlic cloves in olive oil without letting them burn. Take the garlic out, put a clean cotton swab in the warm oil, and insert the swab gently into the ear. This remedy is even mild enough for toddlers.

Another home remedy is to heat kosher salt in a pot, pour it into a clean sock or piece of cheesecloth, and apply it to the ear. The salt draws out the infection and is good for the pain. This is another remedy soothing and gentle enough for toddlers.

A helpful anti-infective internal combination to take for the duration of the problem includes equal parts of:

▼ Echinacea
▼ Goldenseal
▼ Wild indigo

Make a decoction by boiling the three roots in 1½ pints of water for 10 minutes. Reduce to 1 pint. Use 1 ounce of the total combined herbs recommended, and drink up to 3 cups daily. Adding licorice extract or tincture makes the mixture taste better, especially for children.

For infants' ear problems, replace the goldenseal with relaxing hops or chamomile. This remedy can be taken by the mother and is mild enough to pass on to your baby through breast milk.

EMPHYSEMA

Emphysema is a serious, life-threatening disease that requires prompt medical attention. In emphysema, which is almost always caused by cigarette smoking, tiny air sacs in your lungs called alveoli become damaged. This leads to shortness of breath and eventually may cause respiratory or heart failure.

If you choose to complement your medical care with an herbal approach, see a qualified herbal practitioner. Although you can't reverse the damage of emphysema, you may prevent it from getting worse with herbal remedies. A soothing remedy for the bronchial tubes and lungs includes equal parts of three of the following herbs:

▼ Elecampane
▼ Licorice
▼ Coltsfoot
▼ Mullein

Make a decoction by boiling the elecampane and licorice roots in 1½ pints of water for 10 minutes. Reduce to 1 pint. Add the aboveground parts of coltsfoot or mullein, cover, and steep for an additional 10 minutes. Use 1 ounce of the total combined herbs recommended, and drink up to 3 cups daily.

FEVER

Fever, or pyrexia, is a rise in your body's temperature. Fever is a symptom rather than a disease. Most commonly, fevers occur when your body is trying to fight off a viral or bacterial infection. When your body mobilizes white blood cells to fight off infection, proteins called pyrogens are released, causing the body to raise its temperature in yet another attack on the infection.

The goal of herbal remedies is to help your body through its fever in the most efficient way possible. Herbal remedies are often used side by side with antibiotics and other drugs. But unlike drugs such as aspirin, herbal remedies are not intended to simply eliminate your fever. Herbalists see fever as a valuable natural defense against disease. The goal is to shorten the length of your fever and to keep you as comfortable as possible while it runs its course.

A good herbal remedy for fever is ginger tea. You can drink cups of ginger tea all day long; it is diaphoretic, which means it makes you sweat, and it can help you sweat your fever out. Drink plenty of liquids to replace the fluids you lose when you have a fever.

Try taking this helpful herbal combination until your fever breaks:

▼ Elder (2 parts)
▼ Peppermint (1 part)
▼ Yarrow (2 parts)

Make an infusion of the aboveground parts of these herbs. Cover and steep them in 1 pint of hot water for 10 minutes. Use 1 ounce of the total combined herbs recommended, and drink up to 3 cups daily.

FLATULENCE *(Gas)*

Gas is formed in the stomach and bowels by swallowed air or poor diet. Flatulence is the expulsion of gas through the anus; sometimes there is stomach discomfort, which is relieved when gas is expelled.

Charcoal capsules are highly absorbent and can help relieve the discomfort caused by gas. However, avoid using them for a prolonged period of time, as they may cause constipation.

Herbalists look for the background causes of gas. Some cultures offer natural remedies for gas; for example, toasted fennel seeds appear on the tables of many Indian restaurants.

There are many natural carminatives, or herbs that relieve gas and colic in the intestines. They can be brewed as teas, and drunk one to three times daily. Because the carminative herbs are very aromatic, use a little less of them than you would other herbs. An herbal combination for gas might include two or three of the following:

▼ Aniseed
▼ Cardamom
▼ Fennel
▼ Peppermint

All these herbs are used as the aboveground parts of the plants. Make an infusion of two or three of them by putting ¾ teaspoon of the dried herbal combination or 2¼ teaspoons of the fresh into 1 cup of hot water. Cover and steep for 10 minutes. Drink up to 3 cups daily.

The flu, or influenza, is a viral infection that most commonly affects the respiratory tract. There is a sudden onset of fever, chills, intense body aches and pains, and a painful lower-respiratory cough. The flu is spread by infected droplets coughed or sneezed into the air.

Herbal treatment of the flu involves fever management and expectorant remedies, which encourage ridding your lungs of phlegm. Raw garlic is helpful. Ginger tea and peppermint are diaphoretic and will help you sweat out your fever. Goldenseal is useful when there is a respiratory basis to the flu. Boneset can ease the body aches and pains that accompany the flu, while echinacea has both immune-boosting and antibacterial properties.

An herbal combination we recommend for relief of flu symptoms consists of:

- ▼ Echinacea (3 parts)
- ▼ Goldenseal (3 parts)
- ▼ Boneset (3 parts)
- ▼ Peppermint (1 part)

Make a decoction by boiling the echinacea and goldenseal roots in 1½ pints of water for 10 minutes. Reduce to 1 pint. Add the aboveground portions of boneset and peppermint, cover, and steep for an additional 10 minutes. Use 1 ounce of the total combined herbs recommended, and drink up to 3 cups daily.

FOOD POISONING

Food poisoning is an illness caused by eating food that has been contaminated with bacteria. Food poisoning is a severe and life-threatening condition characterized by stomach pain, diarrhea, and vomiting. It requires immediate medical attention.

Herbalism cannot cure food poisoning, but there are herbs you can take to prevent it. Incorporating bitter herbs and hot spices into your diet when you are traveling in unsanitary conditions may help protect you from a bout with food poisoning. Hot, spicy foods naturally increase acidity in the stomach, which may eliminate pathogens before they get into your intestines and cause a serious problem.

When you travel, especially through countries where dysentery is a problem, we suggest that you carry a one-ounce bottle of gentian tincture with you. As a preventive measure, put a couple of drops in your mouth before each meal. Gentian will cause your stomach to become hyperacidic. Bacteria that you may accidentally ingest get killed by the acid in your stomach before they enter your intestines and cause serious trouble.

HAIR LOSS

A receding hairline can send a shiver down the strongest men's spines. Although herbs cannot regenerate new hair growth, they may help prevent premature loss of hair. There are no real cures, but there are a number of time-honored remedies. For example, massaging rosemary oil into your hair before a shampoo can be helpful. A rejuvenating Chinese tonic said to prevent hair from turning gray and falling out is:

▼ Fo-ti

Take 1 to 3 capsules daily.

▲

HAY FEVER

Hay fever, or allergic rhinitis, is triggered by the presence in the air of pollen, dust, mold, or animal hair. Hay fever is an uncomfortable condition: hay fever sufferers experience runny noses, sneezing, and facial pain. Avoiding pollen and other allergens is the logical first step. An herbal combination to relieve hay fever is:

▼ Dandelion root (1 part)

▼ Ephedra (1 part)

▼ Goldenseal (1 part)

▼ Licorice (2 parts)

Make a decoction by boiling the four herbal roots in 1½ pints of water for 10 minutes. Reduce to 1 pint. Use 1 ounce of the total combined herbs, and drink up to 3 cups daily.

HEADACHE

A headache is a very common—but also a very complicated—condition. The trick is to find the reason for the headache. There are many causes for headaches, such as stress, poor diet, overindulgence in alcohol, excessive noise, travel, and poor posture.

Migraine is an especially severe headache, which may be accompanied by nausea and vomiting. Migraine headaches may be triggered by cheese, chocolate, or red wine.

It is important to treat the *causes* of many headaches— for example, those related to digestive problems or stress. When you sort out for yourself where the headaches are coming from, turn to the alphabetical listing of that underlying condition and try the appropriate herbal remedy for it.

Sometimes it is difficult to determine on your own just what is causing your headaches. If you find this to be the case—and your headaches are unusually persistent and do not respond to several days' to a week's home treatment— consult a qualified professional.

For common headaches, a good general relaxant is wood betony.

For migraines, take:

▼ Dandelion (1 part)
▼ Feverfew (2 parts)

Make a decoction by boiling the dandelion root in 1½ pints of water for 10 minutes. Reduce to 1 pint. Add the feverfew leaves, cover, and steep for an additional 10 minutes. Use 1 ounce of the total combined herbs recommended, and drink up to 3 cups daily.

HEART PROBLEMS

Many herbal remedies have a tonic effect upon the heart. Serious heart conditions require medical attention. If you choose to complement your medical care with an herbal approach, see a qualified herbal practitioner.

Many supportive herbal heart remedies can be taken over long periods of time. Hawthorn berry is a good adaptogenic herb; that is, it helps your body adapt to physical, emotional, and environmental stress. Motherwort stabilizes the heart. A helpful heart tonic includes equal parts of:

▼ Hawthorn
▼ Motherwort

Make an infusion of the aboveground parts of hawthorn and motherwort. Cover and steep them in 1 pint of hot water for 10 minutes. Use 1 ounce of the total combined herbs recommended, and drink up to 3 cups daily.

HEMORRHOIDS

Hemorrhoids are varicose veins in the lining of the rectum. Rectal bleeding and pain during bowel movements are the most common symptoms of hemorrhoids. They are very common, especially during and immediately after pregnancy. Lack of exercise and insufficient fiber in your diet can also lead to hemorrhoids.

There are both external and internal herbal treatments for the relief of hemorrhoids. Externally, a soothing and healing ointment of witch hazel is commercially available. Internally, bulk-forming laxatives such as psyllium and flaxseed absorb water in the stool and thereby soften it. An excellent internal combination is composed of equal parts of:

▼ Dandelion
▼ Yellow dock
▼ Horse chestnut

Make a decoction by boiling the dandelion and yellow dock roots in 1½ pints of water for 10 minutes. Reduce to 1 pint. Add the aboveground parts of horse chestnut, cover, and steep for an additional 10 minutes. Use 1 ounce of the total combined herbs, and drink up to 3 cups daily. *Note that pregnant or nursing women should not use this internal remedy.*

HEPATITIS

There are many forms of hepatitis, and all are serious liver diseases that require prompt medical attention. The most common infective types of hepatitis are viral: hepatitis A, which is associated with poor hygiene and diet, and hepatitis B, which is spread mainly through sexual activity and needle sharing among drug users. Hepatitis A is generally less severe than hepatitis B.

Symptoms of hepatitis include jaundice, nausea, vomiting, diarrhea, lack of appetite, and fever. Many people choose to supplement medical treatment with the attention of a qualified herbal practitioner. A helpful herbal combination for hepatitis consists of equal parts of:

▼ Dandelion

▼ Milk thistle

Make a decoction by boiling the dandelion root in 1½ pints of water for 10 minutes. Reduce to 1 pint. Toss in the milk thistle seeds, cover, and steep for an another 10 minutes. Use 1 ounce of the total combined herbs recommended, and drink up to 3 cups daily.

▲

HERPES SIMPLEX

Herpes simplex is a common viral disease that produces cold sores around the mouth and/or blisters on the genitalia. Outbreaks of herpes can be a sign of immunodeficiency or stress. Many people get relief from herpes by taking L-Lysine, an amino acid.

Applied locally, St. John's wort oil or witch hazel may be helpful. Since herpes is so often the result of stress in your life, the following internal combination may prove soothing. Combine equal parts of the herbs and take for the duration of the outbreak:

▼ Dandelion

▼ Echinacea

▼ Licorice

▼ Valerian

Make a decoction by boiling the roots in 1½ pints of water for 10 minutes. Reduce to 1 pint. Use 1 ounce of the total combined herbs recommended, and drink up to 3 cups daily.

HYPERTENSION

Hypertension is an unusually elevated level of blood pressure in your main arteries. Hypertension, or high blood pressure, often goes undetected; yet it can have very serious complications, including heart attack and stroke. High blood pressure requires prompt medical attention.

Reducing salt and excess fat from your diet and engaging in regular aerobic exercise can help reduce mild cases of hypertension. Herbal remedies are also a helpful supplement to conventional medicine. Garlic pills are good for the blood vessels, as they reduce the artery-clogging plaque that often leads to high blood pressure. Dandelion leaves are a mild diuretic, which can help blood circulation. A successful herbal combination consists of:

▼ Hawthorn (2 parts)
▼ Yarrow (1 part)

Make an infusion of the aboveground parts of hawthorn and yarrow. Cover and steep them in 1 pint of hot water for 10 minutes. Use 1 ounce of the total combined herbs recommended, and drink up to 3 cups daily.

INDIGESTION

Indigestion is a digestive disturbance brought on by eating too much food, eating too quickly, or eating food that disagrees with you. Sometimes indigestion can be triggered by stress. The symptoms of indigestion include nausea, vomiting, heartburn, stomach pain, and flatulence.

Po Chai, nicknamed the Chinese Alka-Seltzer, is one

good remedy for indigestion. Ginger tea may be helpful. A combination of the bitter herbs dandelion leaf and gentian can also relieve your indigestion. And yet another herbal combination for occasional bouts of indigestion might include equal parts of any two of the following herbs:

▼ Aniseed
▼ Fennel
▼ Lemon balm

Make an infusion of any two of the three herbs. Cover and steep them in 1 pint of hot water for 10 minutes. Use 1 ounce of the combined herbs, and drink up to 3 cups daily.

Note: If indigestion is chronic, it may indicate a more serious underlying condition, and this should be investigated by a qualified professional.

▲

INFERTILITY

Fertility is the ability to have children without difficulty. A woman's fertile period occurs about halfway through the menstrual cycle. Since sperm can live in a fallopian tube for up to seventy-two hours, there are generally three days during which a woman can get pregnant each cycle.

Before taking herbal combinations to increase fertility, both men and women should make sure that there is nothing medically preventing them from conceiving. There may be a physical problem that needs to be corrected, especially if you have been unsuccessfully trying to conceive for a long period of time.

Herbal combinations to increase fertility should be taken at the rate of 3 cups a day for a period of three months. If you are still experiencing problems after this period, it's best to consult a qualified professional.

An herbal combination to enhance a man's fertility includes:

▼ Asian or Siberian ginseng
▼ Damiana
▼ Saw palmetto

Make a decoction by boiling the ginseng root in 1½ pints of water for 10 minutes. Reduce to 1 pint. Add the aboveground parts of damiana and saw palmetto, cover, and steep for another 10 minutes. Use 1 ounce of the total combined herbs recommended.

Vitamin E may be helpful for a woman's fertility. A beneficial herbal combination for women's fertility problems includes:

▼ Dong quai
▼ False unicorn root
▼ Raspberry

Make a decoction by boiling the dong quai and false unicorn roots in 1½ pints of water for 10 minutes. Reduce to 1 pint. Add the aboveground portion of raspberry leaf, cover, and steep for another 10 minutes. Use 1 ounce of the total combined herbs recommended.

INSOMNIA

From time to time, almost everyone has trouble dropping off to sleep. A common cause of insomnia is worrying about day-to-day problems, such as bills to pay or deadlines to meet at work. Other times, insomnia may be a symptom of a more serious underlying condition, perhaps depression or anxiety. To get a good night's sleep, try sipping a cup of equal parts of this non-habit-forming decoction before bed:

▼ Valerian
▼ Hops

Make a decoction by boiling the valerian root in 1½ pints of water for 10 minutes. Reduce to 1 pint. Add the hops flowers, cover, and steep for an additional 10 minutes. Use 1 ounce of the total combined herbs recommended.

Note: The purpose of this remedy is to make you sleepy, so avoid driving or operating heavy machinery while using it.

LIVER PROBLEMS

The liver is the largest and one of the most important organs in your body. Your liver teams up with your kidneys to rid your body of dangerous toxins, and plays a very important role in regulating the levels of chemicals in your blood.

In the polluted environment in which we live today, our livers have to work very hard to rid our bodies of toxins. There are many herbal remedies that nurture, strengthen, and tone the liver. A gentle detoxifying combination includes equal parts of:

▼ Dandelion
▼ Yellow dock
▼ Milk thistle

Make a decoction by boiling the dandelion and yellow dock roots in 1½ pints of water for 10 minutes. Reduce to 1 pint. Toss in the milk thistle seeds, cover, and steep for an another 10 minutes. Use 1 ounce of the total combined herbs recommended, and drink up to 3 cups daily.

▲

MENOPAUSE

Menopause affects women between the ages of forty-five and fifty-five, as the production of estrogen is drastically reduced and menstruation ceases. Many uncomfortable symptoms accompany menopause. Night sweats and hot flashes are frequent signs of menopause. Women may become irritable or depressed. Weight gain and water retention are also problems.

Herbal remedies are intended to help women proceed through this natural process as smoothly and comfortably as possible. They provide a valuable alternative to hormone-replacement therapy, a common drug treatment that is not appropriate for all women. We recommend the following herbal combination to help ease your passage through menopause:

▼ Dandelion (1 part)
▼ Agnus-castus (2 parts)

▼ Motherwort (1 part)
▼ St. John's wort (1 part)

Make a decoction by boiling the dandelion root in 1½ pints of water for 10 minutes. Reduce to 1 pint. Add the aboveground parts of the other herbs, cover, and steep for an additional 10 minutes. Use 1 ounce of the total combined herbs recommended, and drink 1 to 2 cups a day of this nurturing and supportive herbal combination for intermittent three-month periods.

▲

MENSTRUAL PROBLEMS

Women have menstrual periods beginning in puberty and lasting until menopause. During that time, various problems may arise in the menstrual cycle. Some women experience excessive bleeding; others have irregular periods. And still others endure painful cramps each month.

Individual problems require the attention of a qualified practitioner. But there are many herbs that are particularly suited to the health of the female reproductive system. The following herbal combinations have nurturing and tonic effects that may be helpful to women who suffer from menstrual problems.

For Cramps
▼ Black haw or cramp bark (1 part)
▼ Agnus-castus (2 parts)
▼ Sage (1 part)

Make a decoction by boiling the black haw or cramp bark in 1½ pints of water for 10 minutes. Reduce to 1 pint. Add the agnus-castus berries and sage leaves, cover, and steep for an additional 10 minutes. Use 1 ounce of the total combined herbs recommended, and drink 1 to 3 cups a day for the duration of your problem.

For Irregular Menstrual Periods
- ▼ False unicorn root (2 parts)
- ▼ Agnus-castus (1 part)

Make a decoction by boiling the false unicorn root in 1½ pints of water for 10 minutes. Reduce to 1 pint. Add the agnus-castus berries, cover, and steep for an additional 10 minutes. Use 1 ounce of the total combined herbs recommended, and drink 1 to 3 cups a day for the duration of your problem.

For Excessive Bleeding
- ▼ Agnus-castus (2 parts)
- ▼ Lady's mantle (1 part)

Make an infusion of the agnus-castus berries and lady's mantle. Cover and steep them in 1 pint of hot water for 10 minutes. Use 1 ounce of the total combined herbs recommended, and drink 1 to 3 cups a day for the duration of your problem. If the bleeding is very excessive, 1 part agrimony can also help.

For Scanty Menstrual Periods
- ▼ False unicorn root (2 parts)

▼ Dong quai (1 part)
▼ Agnus-castus (1 part)

Make a decoction by boiling the false unicorn and dong quai roots in 1½ pints of water for 10 minutes. Reduce to 1 pint. Add the agnus-castus berries, cover, and steep for an additional 10 minutes. Use 1 ounce of the total combined herbs recommended, and drink 1 to 3 cups a day for the duration of your problem.

MOTION SICKNESS

Motion sickness can occur in a car, boat, or airplane. Mild cases of motion sickness may involve queasiness and/or headache. More severe cases entail pallor, heavy sweating, vomiting, and an overall feeling of distress.

Studies have shown that ginger is as effective as Dramamine in the relief of motion sickness. The classic herbal remedy for motion sickness is a drop or two of ginger tincture taken before your trip.

NAUSEA

Nausea is a queasy sensation that makes you feel a need to vomit. Nausea may be a symptom of any number of underlying disorders, including motion sickness, stress, stomach problems, and allergic reactions to a food or drug. If there is a serious underlying disorder, it should be identified and treated. In the meantime, try drinking a decoction or infusion made of equal parts of any two or three of these herbs:

▼ Cinnamon
▼ Chamomile
▼ Fennel
▼ Meadowsweet
▼ Peppermint

Cinnamon is a bark, and bark—like roots—must be made into decoctions. Do this by boiling the cinnamon in 1½ pints of water for 10 minutes. Reduce to 1 pint.

The other herbs are aboveground parts of plants and can be made into infusions. Cover and steep them in 1 pint of hot water for 10 minutes. Use 1 ounce of the total combined herbs, and drink up to 3 cups daily.

▲

PAIN

Pain is a sensation in your nerve endings that can range from mild to excruciating. Pain is clearly the symptom of an injury or disease, which likewise may be very mild or very serious. Once the underlying problem is identified and treated, there are a number of natural anesthetics that may be appropriate as adjunctive treatments.

Meadowsweet and white willow bark are known as herbal aspirins. Both herbs contain the active chemical salicin, from which the first aspirin was actually made. Salicin has natural pain-reducing, fever-reducing, and anti-inflammatory properties. Valerian is a natural relaxant, which makes pain more tolerable. A natural combination to relieve mild pain includes equal parts of the following herbs:

▼ Meadowsweet
▼ Valerian
▼ White willow

Make a decoction by boiling the valerian and white willow bark in 1½ pints of water for 10 minutes. Reduce to 1 pint. Add the aboveground parts of meadowsweet, cover, and steep for an additional 10 minutes. Use 1 ounce of the combined herbs recommended, and drink up to 3 cups daily.

▲

PALPITATIONS

Palpitations are a feeling of fluttering or thumping in the chest. They are usually not serious, but may be very frightening. Palpitations are brought on by a number of causes, such as stress, a frightening experience, indigestion, heavy smoking, or overindulgence in alcohol or caffeine.

To be safe, you should consult a qualified professional if you have palpitations, especially if they persist or are accompanied by chest pain. A helpful herbal combination for palpitations includes:

▼ Hawthorn (2 parts)
▼ Motherwort (1 part)

Make an infusion of the hawthorn and motherwort. Cover and steep them in 1 pint of hot water for 10 minutes.

Use 1 ounce of the combined herbs, and drink up to·3 cups daily.

Note: If palpitations are accompanied by anxiety, add 1 part of valerian or hops to the formula. Hawthorn should remain the primary ingredient.

▲

POISON IVY

Poison ivy, poison oak, and poison sumac are common poisonous plants that can cause severe allergic reactions if they brush against your skin. Itching, burning, and blistering occur in varying degrees, according to an individual's sensitivity.

First aid for poison ivy is to wash the area thoroughly with soap and water. Bathe the area with vinegar or apply chickweed ointment to relieve the itch. Epsom salts or oatmeal baths may also provide some comfort. Internally, try drinking a combination of equal parts of chaparral and echinacea:

▼ Echinacea
▼ Chaparral

Make a decoction by boiling the echinacea root in 1½ pints of water for 10 minutes. Reduce to 1 pint. Add the aboveground parts of chaparral, cover, and steep for an additional 10 minutes. Use 1 ounce of the combined herbs recommended, and drink up to 3 cups daily.

PMS *(Premenstrual Syndrome)*

Many women experience uncomfortable physical and emotional symptoms a week or two before menstruation; this is known as PMS, or premenstrual syndrome. Physical symptoms most commonly include water retention, breast tenderness, and lower-back pain. Emotionally, many women experience mood swings, irritability, tension, and fatigue. A helpful herbal combination may include:

- ▼ Black haw (1 part)
- ▼ Agnus-castus (2 parts)
- ▼ Motherwort (1 part)

Make a decoction by boiling the black haw bark in 1½ pints of water for 10 minutes. Reduce to 1 pint. Add the aboveground parts of agnus-castus and motherwort, cover, and steep for an additional 10 minutes. Use 1 ounce of the combined herbs recommended. Begin taking this herbal combination right after ovulation and continue through the beginning of your period. Drink 1 to 3 cups a day.

Note: Other herbs can be added to relieve additional symptoms.

▲

PROSTATE PROBLEMS

Serious prostate problems, such as cancer, require immediate medical attention. A more benign prostate problem —enlargement—happens to almost all men as they grow older. Urinary retention, reduced urinary flow, difficulty in urination, frequent urination, and incontinence are all possible symptoms of prostate enlargement.

Severe cases of prostate enlargement require the attention of a qualified professional. Mild symptoms may respond to treatment with equal parts of these herbs:

▼ Damiana
▼ Horsetail
▼ Saw palmetto

Make an infusion of aboveground parts of these herbs. Cover and steep them in 1 pint of hot water for 10 minutes. Use 1 ounce of the combined herbs, and drink up to 3 cups daily.

▲

PSORIASIS

Psoriasis is a common skin disease characterized by patches of thickened red skin. Qualified herbalists may search for the underlying toxic causes of psoriasis. External relief may come from oil of St. John's wort or comfrey lotion or ointment. An internal combination for the relief of symptoms includes equal parts of:

▼ Burdock
▼ Dong quai
▼ Echinacea
▼ Yellow dock

Make a decoction by boiling the herbs in 1½ pints of water for 10 minutes. Reduce to 1 pint. Use 1 ounce of the total combined herbs recommended, and drink up to 3 cups daily.

SORE THROAT

A sore throat is a symptom of an underlying ailment, such as a cold, flu, laryngitis, tonsillitis, and a variety of viral infections. If the underlying condition is serious, it requires prompt professional treatment.

Sore throats may be soothed with both gargles and systemic remedies. Swallowing a small amount of finely minced garlic and honey is very healing, although it may burn a little. Gargling with a few drops of tincture of myrrh mixed with water is also helpful. Internally, sore throats can be treated like a cold. Herbal relief for sore throats includes equal parts of:

▼ Elder
▼ Peppermint
▼ Yarrow

Make an infusion of aboveground parts of these herbs. Cover and steep them in 1 pint of hot water for 10 minutes. Use 1 ounce of the total combined herbs, and drink up to 3 cups daily.

STRESS

Stress is an anxious feeling, which may be in response to major life events, such as the death of a spouse, or it may be due to difficulty in coping with the simple aggravations of day-to-day life. Stress should not be taken lightly: continuous stress can lead to serious conditions such as high blood pressure, depression, lowered immune function, and even certain types of cancer.

Exercise is one natural remedy we can all use to reduce stress. It's also very important to understand and deal with the underlying causes of your stress. In the meantime, a soothing herbal combination contains equal parts of:

▼ Valerian

▼ Damiana

▼ Hops

Make a decoction by boiling the valerian root in 1½ pints of water for 10 minutes. Reduce to 1 pint. Add the aboveground parts of damiana and hops, cover, and steep for an additional 10 minutes. Use 1 ounce of the total combined herbs recommended, and drink up to 3 cups daily.

This remedy makes some people sleepy, so avoid driving or operating heavy machinery while using it. While you may drink up to 3 cups a day, begin with 1 cup after dinner and gradually increase your dosage as needed.

An alternative herbal remedy for stress—one that will not make you so sleepy—includes:

▼ Damiana (1 part)

▼ Valerian (or passionflower) (1 part)

▼ Vervain (2 parts)

Make an infusion of the aboveground parts of damiana, valerian (or passionflower), and vervain. Cover and steep them in 1 pint of hot water for 10 minutes. Use 1 ounce of the total combined herbs, and drink up to 3 cups daily.

SUNBURN

Sunburn is an inflammation of the skin due to overexposure to the sun. Repeated sunburns over time may cause premature aging of your skin and increased risk of skin cancer. Try to be sensible about exposure to the sun. Fair-skinned people should exercise special caution: be sure to use plenty of sunscreen with an SPF of at least 15, and limit periods of tanning.

If you do get a sunburn, vinegar can help take the sting out. The classic restorative herbal remedy for sunburn is aloe vera gel, applied locally as needed.

TOOTH AND GUM PROBLEMS

Regular tooth care is an important part of your overall hygiene, and herbs can play a role in both preventing decay and relieving painful tooth and gum aches. Clove oil, for example, is an active ingredient in many over-the-counter preparations, such as Lavoris mouthwash. Myrrh can help kill the bacteria that lead to tooth decay, and a toothpaste called Merfluan is available in many health food stores.

Serious toothaches require professional care. In the meantime, helpful external herbal tinctures to dab on a cotton swab and apply to your toothache are:

▼ Clove
▼ Myrrh

Apply locally as needed.

URINARY-TRACT INFECTIONS

Urinary-tract infections (UTIs), which primarily affect women, are usually characterized by painful and frequent urination. Large quantities of liquid should be drunk; alcohol should be avoided. If the condition persists, or if you think it might be the result of a sexually transmitted disease, see your medical doctor.

A natural remedy for urinary-tract infections is to drink plenty of cranberry juice; make sure the juice is from a health food store, not the sugary kind you find in most supermarkets. Taking 5 to 6 grams of vitamin C each day may also help. If your infection still doesn't get better, an internal urinary disinfectant herbal combination might include:

▼ Buchu (1 part)
▼ Corn silk (2 parts)
▼ Juniper or uva-ursi (1 part)

Make an infusion of the aboveground parts of buchu, corn silk, and juniper or uva-ursi. (Corn silk, a mucilaginous healing remedy for the urinary tract, can be taken off corn when you shuck it; you can also use the water corn was cooked in.) Cover and steep them in 1 pint of hot water for 10 minutes. Use 1 ounce of the total combined herbs, and drink up to 3 cups daily. If your infection does not clear up within a week or so, seek professional help.

Note: Do not use this internal formula if you are experiencing any pain in the kidney area. It can be aggravating to the kidneys.

VARICOSE VEINS

Varicose veins usually occur on the back of the calf and on the insides of your legs. More common in women than in men, serious cases of varicose veins require medical attention. Swollen veins become blue and are sometimes prominently raised. Conditions that aggravate varicose veins are obesity, constipation, standing for long periods of time, and pregnancy.

Exercise and raising the legs whenever possible may help relieve the pain of varicose veins. Externally, St. John's wort oil, marigold ointment, or a witch hazel compress may help. Cayenne and ginger are useful because they keep peripheral circulation alive. If your bowels are plugged up, pressure is added to your veins; so if you are also constipated, add a bulk laxative such as psyllium to your treatment. An internal combination for varicose veins contains equal parts of the following herbs:

▼ Dandelion root
▼ Witch hazel
▼ Yellow dock

Make a decoction by boiling the three herbs in 1½ pints of water for 10 minutes. Reduce to 1 pint. Use 1 ounce of the total combined herbs recommended, and drink up to 3 cups daily. Nursing and pregnant women should not use this remedy.

WHOOPING COUGH

Whooping cough, or pertussis, is a distressing infection that primarily affects young children. Bouts of coughing lead to breathlessness and the characteristic *whoop*. Whooping cough should be treated by qualified practitioners. A helpful herbal combination includes equal parts of:

▼ Licorice
▼ Wild cherry bark
▼ Coltsfoot
▼ Thyme

Make a decoction by boiling the licorice root and wild cherry bark in 1½ pints of water for 10 minutes. Reduce to 1 pint. Add the aboveground parts of coltsfoot and thyme, cover, and steep for an additional 10 minutes. Use 1 ounce of the total combined herbs recommended, and drink up to 3 cups daily. (See page 208 for precautions concerning wild cherry bark.)

▲

WOUNDS

Minor cuts and scrapes respond well to herbal treatment, while serious wounds require immediate medical attention. First stop the bleeding by applying pressure. An excellent Chinese patent remedy for bleeding, available in Chinese pharmacies, is Yunnan Pai Yao. The powder of Yunnan Pai Yao can be applied to cuts and abrasions—that is, open cuts that are not very serious. Carefully follow the directions on any commercial remedy.

Rinse minor wounds under cold running water and

gently wipe with antiseptic cotton or gauze. Vitamin E can also be used to help prevent scarring. Before securing the wound with a sterile bandage, try applying one of these herbal remedies:

▼ Calendula ointment
▼ St. John's wort oil

Apply locally as needed.

▲
YEAST INFECTIONS

Yeast infections, or candidiasis, is caused by a fungus. Yeast infections often occur in the vaginal area, although they may also develop in the mouth (where they are usually known as thrush). Yeast infections occur in both men and women and can be passed on through sexual intercourse. A vaginal yeast infection is characterized by a thick, white discharge; a woman may also experience intense irritation and itching. Men may experience inflammation of the head of the penis. Antifungal drugs are used to clear up yeast infections.

It's helpful to cut down on dairy products and refined carbohydrates and to eliminate alcohol and caffeine during the course of your treatment. A vaginal douche made with echinacea and pau d'arco can be used three times each week. We also recommend this helpful herbal combination:

▼ Dandelion
▼ Echinacea
▼ Pau d'arco
▼ Cleavers

Make a decoction by boiling the dandelion root, echinacea root, and pau d'arco bark in 1½ pints of water for 10 minutes. Reduce to 1 pint. Add the aboveground parts of cleavers, cover, and steep for an additional 10 minutes. Use 1 ounce of the total combined herbs recommended, and drink up to 3 cups daily.

INDEX

Aaron's rod, 176
Acne, 214, 221–222
Adderwort, 68
Adenoid problems, 91
Aerobic exercise, 10, 20, 28,
    29
Agnus-castus (*Vitex agnus-
    castus*), 38, 47–48,
    260–263, 267
Agrimony (*Agrimonia
    eupatoria*), 48–49, 242
AIDS (Acquired Immune
    Deficiency Syndrome),
    2, 30, 61, 132, 191,
    192, 194, 195, 214,
    220, 222–223
Alcohol consumption, 8, 9,
    28, 31–33, 35, 40, 232,
    243, 275
Alfafa (*Medicago sativa*), 50–
    51
Allantoin, 97, 201
Allergic reactions, 20, 52–53,
    88, 117, 123, 182
Almond (*Prunus amygdalus*),
    51–53
Aloe vera (*Aloe barbadenis*),
    11, 53–54, 229, 271

American Association of
    Naturopathic
    Physicians, 21
American Botanical Council,
    21
American ginseng (*Panax
    quinquefolium*), 140–
    142
American Herb Association,
    21
Ames, Bruce, 99
Anemia, 50, 55, 110, 215
Angelica (*Angelica
    archangelica*), 36, 55–
    56, 99
Anger, 6, 33, 40
Angina, 154
Animal protein, 8, 9
Aniseed (*Pimpinella anisum*),
    11, 36, 37, 56–57,
    257
Anorexia, 73, 85
Anthraquinones, 214
Antibiotics, 30, 34, 35, 66,
    89, 112, 131–133, 149,
    150, 231, 247
Antioxidants, 27, 30, 89, 90,
    105, 106

Antiseptics, 93, 120, 159, 199–201

Anxiety, 9, 32, 40, 121, 129, 163, 175, 195, 211, 212, 266

Aphrodisiacs, 39, 104, 130, 143, 196, 197

Apiole, 183

Appetite, 73, 85, 116, 134, 135, 141, 144

Arbutin, 201

Arnica (*Arnica montana*), 58–59, 80

Arthritis, 51, 58, 70, 72, 78, 79, 85, 107, 113, 114, 117, 120, 121, 127, 135, 137, 158, 160, 162, 166, 168, 172, 206, 223–224

Artichoke (*Cynara scolymus*), 59–60

Asian ginseng (*Panax ginseng*), 140, 141, 143–145, 258

Asiaticoside, 151

Asparagine, 50

Asparagus root (*Asparagus officinalis*), 60–62

Aspirin, 71, 73, 171–172, 206, 207

Asthma, 70, 72, 95, 100, 115–117, 139, 167, 168, 177, 182, 197, 200, 208, 220, 224–225

Astragalus (*Astralagus membranaceous*), 2, 30–31, 39, 62–63, 222

Atherosclerosis, 60, 154

Athlete's foot, 49, 150, 184, 225–226

Atonic constipation, 237

Aucubin, 187

Australian gum, 119

Autoimmune diseases, 30

Azulene, 212

Back pain, 50, 87

Bad breath, 57, 93, 109, 126, 179, 183, 220, 226–227

Balm of Gilead (*Populus gileadensis), 36, 64*

Barberry (*Berberis vulgaris*), 39, 65–66

Bardane, 77

Bayberry (*Myrica cerifera*), 17, 66–67, 123

Beans, 26, 32, 33

Bearberry, 201

Bed-wetting, 76

Beggar's-buttons, 77

Berberine, 149

Beta-carotene, 31, 50

Betony, 211

Bicycling, 10

Bile flow, 17

Biofeedback, 41

Bistort (*Polygonum bistorta*), 68–69

Black cohosh (*Cimicifuga racemosa*), 69–71, 99
Black haw (*Viburnum prunifolium*), 38, 71–73, 99, 261, 267
Black snakeroot, 69
Bladder problems, 87, 90, 132, 159
Bleeding, 49, 73, 81, 98, 100, 102, 103, 161, 210
Blessed thistle (*Cnicus benedictus*), 73–74
Bloating, 50, 57, 61, 91, 183, 202
Blood pressure, 28, 29, 72, 105, 106, 111, 118, 132, 145, 153
Bloodwort, 212
Blue gum, 119
Boils, 78, 198
Boneset (*Eupatorium perfoliatum*), 74–75, 249
Bottlebrush, 157
Breathing, 36–37
Bridewort, 171
Bronchitis, 57, 70, 84, 85, 95, 112, 115, 117, 119, 127, 132, 136, 149, 150, 167, 168, 177, 187, 191, 192, 197, 200, 208, 227–228
Bruises, 58, 90, 114, 168,

171, 195, 196, 213, 228–229
Buchu (*Barosma betulina*) or (*Agathosma betulina*), 76–77, 272
Buckthorn, 82
Bugbane, 69
Burdock (*Arctium lappa*), 39, 77–79, 268
Burns, 18, 53, 54, 80, 81, 92, 102, 103, 113, 114, 152, 170, 171, 195, 196, 198, 229
Butcher's-broom (*Ruscus aculeatus*), 79–80

Caffeine, 15, 35, 40, 225, 232, 275
Calcium, 50, 224
Calendula (*Calendula officinalis*), 80–81, 226, 229, 275
Camphor, 212, 234
Cancer, 2, 6, 8, 9, 11, 50, 89, 97, 98, 112, 132, 144, 166, 184, 185, 191, 192, 214, 220, 229–230
Candleberry, 66
Candlewick, 176
Canker sores, 78, 179
Capsules, 16–17
Carbohydrates, 9, 275
Carbon dioxide, 36

Cardamom seeds, 32, 33, 226, 227, 243, 248

Carminatives, 248

Carosella, 125

Carvacrol, 199

Cascara sagrada (*Rhamnus purshiana*), 82–83, 237

Catnip (*Nepeta cataria*), 83–84

Cayenne (*Capsicum frutescens*), 85–86, 273

Chamomile (*Matricaria chamomilla*), 1, 32, 33, 42, 83, 87–88, 236, 238, 244, 245, 264

Chaparral (*Larrea tridentata*), 11, 89–91, 266

Charcoal capsules, 248

Chasteberry, 47

Chaste tree, 47

Chemotherapy, 53, 63, 136

Cholesterol, 28–30, 50, 52, 60, 126–127, 132, 137, 141, 144, 179, 189, 230–231

Chronic fatigue, 61, 231–232

Chymopapain, 181

Cinnamon, 264

Cinnamon bark, 49

Circulation, 79, 138, 139, 151, 152, 193

Cirrhosis of the liver, 21, 232–233

Cleavers (*Galium aparine*), 91–92, 221, 224, 226, 235, 275–276

Clivers, 91

Cloves (*Caryophyllus aromaticus*), 1, 93–94, 271

Cocklebur, 48

Coffee, 32, 34

Colds, 55–57, 84, 85, 90, 109, 112, 114, 119, 120, 123, 125, 127, 132, 133, 136, 163–165, 172, 176, 177, 185, 186, 197–200, 204, 208, 213, 220, 233–234

Cold sores, 166, 234–235, 255

Colic, 1, 56, 57, 87, 108, 109, 125, 136, 163, 164, 180, 183, 186, 235–236

Colitis, 68, 82, 102, 150, 198, 208

Coltsfoot (*Tussilago farfara*), 36, 37, 64, 70, 94–96, 228, 239, 240, 246, 274

Comfrey (*Symphytum officinale*), 97–99, 268

Companion Plants, 22

Compresses, 18

Conjunctivitis, 123, 125, 126, 150, 170, 171, 236–237

Constipation, 7, 10, 33, 34, 50, 53, 75, 82, 111, 188, 189, 214, 237–238

Convalescence, 50, 140, 143, 146, 211
Convulsions, 168
Corn silk, 272
Cortisone, 107
Coughs, 55, 57, 64, 70, 85, 94, 95, 109, 115, 116, 125, 127, 165, 167, 168, 176, 177, 187, 191, 192, 197–200, 208, 238–240
Coughwort, 94
Cow clover, 191
Cramp bark (*Viburnum opulus*), 28, 71, 99–100, 168, 224
Cramps, menstrual, 55, 61, 69, 70–72, 80, 81, 87, 99, 100, 129, 137, 161, 172, 175, 195, 200, 201, 203, 206, 207, 213, 261–262
Cranberry (*Vaccinium macrocarpon*), 28, 101–102, 272
Cranesbill (*Geranium maculatum*), 102–103
Creams, 18
Crohn's disease, 242
Cystitis, 50, 76, 92, 157

Damiana (*Turnera aphrodisiaca*) or (*diffusa*), 38, 39, 41, 103–105, 232, 240, 258, 268, 270
Dandelion (*Taraxacum officinale*), 2, 28, 29, 31–35, 42, 105–107, 221, 226, 227, 230, 232, 233, 242, 243, 251, 252, 254–257, 260, 273, 275–276
Decoctions, 12–14
Deep breathing, 41
Depression, 156, 162, 164, 180, 195, 240
Devil's-claw (*Harpagophytum procumbens*), 107–108, 224
Diabetes mellitus, 17, 19, 20, 56, 60, 62, 66, 67, 76, 87, 116, 130, 133, 139, 141, 144, 147–149, 184, 220, 241, 242
Diarrhea, 1, 5, 10, 66, 68, 90, 102, 149, 150, 161, 172, 176, 177, 179, 186, 187, 190, 198, 200, 201, 208, 242
Diet, 6, 8, 9, 26, 28–33, 243
Diet pills, 117
Digestion, 17, 32–34, 56, 57, 65, 67, 68, 73, 82, 93, 108, 109, 125, 130, 132–136, 149, 150, 154, 155, 163, 172, 179, 181, 182, 184–

Digestion (*cont.*)
186, 188, 192, 193,
198, 206, 208, 212,
213, 243–244
Dill (*Anethum graveolens*),
108–110
Diuretics, 20, 29, 35, 61, 63,
105, 106, 158–160,
183, 201–203
Diverticulitis, 68
Dizziness, 244
Doctor of Naturopathy, 20
Dong quai (*Angelica
senensis*), 39, 110–111,
258, 263, 268
Douches, 17–18
Dragon weed, 68
Drug abuse, 35, 40
Drug withdrawal, 180
Dysentery, 67, 68, 102, 134,
250

Ear problems, 80, 81, 133,
134, 149, 150, 245
East-West Herb Products, 23
Echinacea (*Echinacea
angustifolia*), 2, 18, 30–
31, 111–113, 221, 223,
226, 230, 232, 234–
236, 245, 249, 255,
266, 268, 275–276
Eczema, 78, 90, 113, 121,
150, 166, 191, 192

Elder (*Sambucus nigra*), 43,
114–115, 234, 247, 269
Elecampane (*Inula helenium*),
1, 36, 37, 115–116,
168, 225, 227, 239, 246
Eleutherosides, 146
Emphysema, 95, 115, 117,
177, 200, 246
English serpentary, 68
Enteritis, 198
Environmental pollutants, 25
Ephedra (*Ephedra sinica*),
116–119, 225, 251
Ephedrine, 118
Estrogen, 123, 127, 145, 192
Eucalyptol, 119, 120
Eucalyptus (*Eucalyptus
globulus*), 119–120
Eugenol, 93, 212
Evening primrose (*Oenothera
biennis*), 121–122
Exercise, 6–10, 20, 28, 29, 37,
40, 270
Extracts, 16
Eye ailments, 122–123
Eyebright (*Euphrasia
officinalis*), 122–123,
236

Flase unicorn root
(*Chamaelirium luteum*),
38, 39, 71, 99, 123–
125, 258, 262
Fat, 8, 9, 28, 29

Fatigue, chronic, 231–232
Featherfew, 128
Feltwort, 176
Fennel (*Foeniculum vulgare*), 42, 43, 123, 125–126, 226, 227, 248, 257, 264
Fenugreek (*Trigonella foenumgraecum*), 32, 33, 126–128, 243
Fertility, 38–39, 61, 124, 130, 196, 197, 257–258
Feverfew (*Tanacetum parthenium*), 128–130, 219, 244, 252
Fevers, 55, 66, 72–76, 80, 81, 84, 88, 92, 133, 149, 168, 172, 173, 185, 204–205, 209, 213, 246–247
Feverwort, 74
Fiber, 8, 26, 30, 32, 33, 237, 238
Fibroid tumors, 47
Finocchio, 125
Fish, 30
Flatulence (gas), 11, 55–57, 73, 82, 85, 93, 108, 109, 125, 133–135, 164, 183, 186, 204, 248
Flavonoids, 194
Flaxseed, 254
Fleaseed, 188
Flu, 55, 74, 75, 90, 109, 112, 114, 119, 120, 132, 133, 136, 149, 150, 163–165, 172, 185, 186, 249
Folic acid, 31, 40
Food additives, 26
Food and Drug Administration (FDA), 2–3, 21, 98, 181
Food poisoning, 67, 132, 135, 168, 169, 193, 242, 250
Fo-ti (*Polygonum multiflorum*), 130–131, 151, 251
Fruits, 8, 9, 30–33, 243

Galegine, 148
Gallbladder problems, 17, 65, 108, 170, 214
Gammalinolenic acid (GLA), 121
Ganoderma fungus, 222
Garlic (*Allium sativum*), 131–134, 226, 231, 245, 249, 256
Gas (*see* Flatulence (gas))
Gastrin, 17
Gastritis, 67, 80, 81, 150, 198, 208
Geneva, 159
Genistein, 191
Gentian (*Gentiana lutea*), 1, 32, 33, 134–135, 226, 227, 235, 241, 243, 250, 257

Ginger (*Zingiber officinale*), 11, 67, 99, 114, 136–137, 239, 244, 247, 249, 257, 263, 273

Gingivitis, 179, 209

Ginkgo (*Ginkgo biloba*), 138–140

Ginseng, 38, 39, 151, 231, 241
    American (*Panax quinquefolium*), 140–142
    Asian (*Panax ginseng*), 140, 141, 143–145, 258
    Siberian (*Eleutherococcus senticosus*), 140, 141, 145–147, 258

Ginsenosides, 140–141, 143, 146

Glycosides, 153

Goat's rue (*Galega officinalis*), 148–149, 241

Goldenseal (*Hydrastis canadensis*), 39, 65, 123, 149–151, 223, 227, 234, 245, 249, 251

Goose grass, 91

Gotu kola (*Centella asiatica*), 151–153

Gout, 107, 157, 159

Grains, 8, 9, 30–33, 40

Greasewood, 89

Green Terrestrial, 23

Guar gum, 241

Gums (*see* Tooth and gum problems)

Gum tree, 119

Hair loss, 250–251

Hansen's disease, 151, 152

Harpagoside, 107

Harvard Medical School, 4

Hawthorn (*Crataegus oxyacantha*), 27–29, 153–155, 231, 253, 256, 265, 266

Hay fever, 114, 117, 149, 150, 177, 251

Headache, 5, 7, 10, 72, 117, 128, 129, 162, 193, 196, 205, 206, 211, 212, 219, 252

Health Center for Better Living, 23

Heart, 1, 6, 9, 27–29, 62, 132, 138, 139, 146, 153, 154, 175, 202, 253

Heartburn, 55, 135, 172, 186

Helonias root, 123

Hemorrhoids, 48, 49, 67, 78, 79, 82, 102, 156, 157, 171, 176, 177, 187, 210, 211, 214, 253–254

Hepatitis, 35, 65, 73, 254–255

Herbalists, locating qualified, 20–21

Herb and Spice Collection, The, 23
Herbe militaire, 212
Herb-of-the-cross, 204
HerbPharm's Whole Herb Catalog, 23
Herpes simplex, 90, 164, 166, 195, 220, 234, 255
High blood pressure (*see* Hypertension)
Hives, 8
HIV (human immunodeficiency virus), 191, 192, 194, 195, 214, 222–223
Hops (*Humulus lupulus*), 32, 33, 41, 155–156, 244, 245, 259, 266, 270
Horse chestnut (*Aesculus hippocastanum*), 156–157, 228, 254
Horsefly weed, 209
Horseheal, 115
Horse hoof, 94
Horsetail (*Equisetum arvense*), 42, 157–159, 268
House dust, 37
Humidifiers, 37
Humulus, 155
Hydrastine, 149
Hydrocyanic acid, 208
Hyperactivity, 83, 84
Hypericin, 194
Hypertension, 28, 62, 70, 72, 105, 106, 111, 118, 121, 129, 132, 145, 153, 154, 202, 213, 256
Hypoglycemia, 130
Hysteria, 100, 168

Immune system, 2, 26, 30–31, 63, 65, 112, 141, 143, 149, 150, 151
Impotence, 124
Indian elm, 198
Indian pennywort, 151
Indigestion, 55, 75, 85, 87, 125, 129, 133, 136, 155, 164, 170, 200, 256–257
Infertility, 124, 257–258
Infusions, 13, 14
Insect bites, 48, 49, 168, 187
Insomnia, 70, 84, 87, 111, 155, 175, 186, 220, 259
Insulin, 17, 25–27, 78
Iron, 50, 78, 215
Irritable-bowel syndrome, 242
Isatis, 222–223

Jacobs, Joe, 4–5
Jaundice, 65, 73, 75, 82, 215
Jaundice berry, 65
Juniper (*Juniperus communis*), 39, 159–161, 272

Kava, 39
Kegel exercises, 40

Kidneys, 34–35, 60, 73, 77, 87, 130, 159, 160, 202, 272
Kidney stones, 61, 92
Knitbone, 97

Labor pains, 69, 70
Lady's foxglove, 176
Lady's mantle (*Alchemilla vulgaris*) and (*xanthochlora*), 43, 161–162, 262
Lapacho, 184
Lappa, 77
Laprachol, 184
Laryngitis, 64, 161, 200, 209
Lavender (*Lavandula officinalis*), 42, 162–163
Lead, 133
Legumes, 31
Lemon balm (*Melissa officinalis*), 32, 33, 43, 83, 163–165, 236, 244, 257
Leonurine, 175
Leopard's bane, 58
Leprosy, 151
Lice, 56, 57
Licorice (*Glycyrrhiza glabra*), 36, 37, 165–167, 223, 225, 227, 228, 239, 240, 246, 251, 255, 274
Life expectancy, 25–26
Lifestyle, 6, 8–10, 25, 26

Liver, 2 17, 34–35, 53, 65, 82, 96, 99, 108, 130, 142, 144, 173–174, 214, 232–233, 259–260
Lobelia (*Lobelia inflata*), 36, 37, 167–170, 225, 239
Lobeline, 169
Longevity, 130, 151, 152
Lucerne, 50
Lungwort, 176
Lymphatic system, 91, 209

Magnesium, 50, 224
Maidenhair tree, 138
Mail order sources, 22–24
Marigold (*Calendula officinalis*), 170–171, 236, 273
Marsh pennywort, 151
Maybloom, 153
Mayflower, 153
Meadowsweet (*Filipendula ulmaria*) or (*Spiraea ulmaria*), 171–173, 206, 224, 242, 264, 265
Meditation, 41
Melon tree, 181
Memory, 138, 141, 144, 193
Meningitis, 112
Menopause, 47, 49, 87, 100, 110, 126, 143, 145, 161, 175, 180, 192, 195, 260–261

Menstrual problems
    cramps, 55, 61, 69, 70–72,
        80, 81, 87, 99, 100,
        129, 137, 161, 172,
        175, 195, 200, 201,
        203, 206, 207, 213,
        261–262
    excessive bleeding, 100,
        102, 161, 262
    irregular cycles, 73–74,
        110, 124, 170, 171,
        175, 179, 183, 194, 262
    PMS (premenstrual
        syndrome), 47, 100,
        105, 106, 110, 121,
        175, 183, 203
    scanty, 262–263
2-methyl-3-butene-2-ol, 155
Midsummer daisy, 128
Migraine headache, 128, 129,
    193, 219, 252
Milk thistle (*Silybum
    marianum*), 2, 34, 173–
    174, 233, 255, 260
Miscarriage, 71, 72, 124
Mold spores, 37
Monk's pepper, 47
Morning sickness, 124, 136
Motherwort (*Leonurus
    cardiaca*), 28, 29, 175–
    176, 253, 261, 265, 267
Motion sickness, 11, 136, 263
Mouthwash, 17
Mucilage, 95, 176, 188, 198

Mucus, 10, 36
Mullein (*Verbascum thapsus*),
    36, 37, 176–178, 228,
    239, 240, 246
Mumps, 137
Muscle spasms, 28, 55, 99,
    100, 172
Myricitrin, 66
Myristicin, 183
Myrrh (*Commiphora myrrha*),
    1, 17, 178–179, 226,
    234, 269, 271

National Institutes of Health
    (NIH), 4
Nature's Herbs, 23
Nausea, 11, 20, 57, 134–137,
    140, 172, 186, 263–264
Nettle, 42
Neuralgia, 69, 70
*New England Journal of
    Medicine, The*, 4, 137
Nicotine addiction, 168
Nipples, sore, 209
Nordihydroguaiaretic acid
    (NDGA), 89, 90
Nosebleed, 213
Nursing, 1, 19, 47, 51, 57, 61,
    74, 79, 91, 96, 99, 108,
    118, 125, 127, 148,
    154, 156, 164, 167,
    169, 174, 194, 202,
    209, 235, 245, 254, 273

Oats (*Avena sativa*), 180–181, 240
Oils, 18
Ointments, 18
Omega-3 fatty acids, 29–30
Organ transplants, 139
Oxygen, 36

Pain, 72, 172, 205, 206, 264–265
Palpitations, 100, 118, 154, 175, 180, 265–266
Panic attacks, 203
Papain, 181
Papaw, 181
Papaya (*Carica papaya*), 181–182
Parasitic infections, 184, 185
Parsley (*Petroselinum sativum*), 43, 183–184
Passive smoke, 36, 37, 174
Pasteur, Louis, 25
Pau d'arco (*Tabebuia heptaphylla*), 18, 184–185, 275–276
Penicillin, 3, 131
Pennyroyal, 39
Peppermint (*Mentha piperita*), 42, 114, 185–187, 234, 247, 248, 249, 264, 269
Pepsin, 181
Pesticides, 26
Pewterwort, 157
Phenylbutazone, 107

Phlebitis, 58, 157
Phyto-Pharmica, 23
Pills, 16–17
Pinkeye, 236
Planetary Formulas, 24
Plantago, 188
Plantain (*Plantago major*), 187–188, 228
Platelet activity factor (PAF), 138, 139
PMS (premenstrual syndrome), 47, 100, 105, 106, 110, 121, 175, 183, 203, 267
Po Chai, 256
Poison ivy and oak, 78, 168, 266
Pollen, 37
Polyacetylenes, 77
Potassium, 35, 50, 106, 158, 159, 203, 242
Poultices, 18
Pregnancy, 19, 38–40, 48, 54, 56, 66, 69–74, 79, 81, 83, 91, 96, 99, 100, 108, 109, 111, 118, 122, 128, 129, 135, 136, 148, 151, 154, 159, 160, 162, 167, 169, 171, 175, 176, 179, 182, 189, 190, 194, 201, 202, 207, 208, 254, 273

Premenstrual syndrome (*see*
      PMS (premenstrual
      syndrome))
Prevention, 8–10
Progesterone, 47
Prostaglandins, 121, 122, 206
Prostate problems, 50, 76,
      157, 158, 196, 197,
      267–268
Pseudo Ginseng, 231
Psoriasis, 78, 91, 92, 113,
      152, 192, 195, 196,
      214, 220, 268
Psyllium (*Plantago psyllium*),
      188–189, 237, 253, 273
Purple clover, 191
Purple coneflower, 111
Pyrogens, 247
Pyrrolizide alkaloids, 96

Queen of the meadow, 171

Radiation burns, 53, 54
Rainbow Light, 24
Raspberry (*Rubus idaeus*), 39,
      190–191, 258
Rattleroot, 69
Reaction time, 138
Red clover (*Trifolium
      pratense*), 2, 11, 30–31,
      89, 191–192, 223, 230
Red elm, 198
Reichi mushroom, 222

Reproductive system, 38–40,
      61, 72, 123, 124
Respiratory problems, 1, 36–
      37, 64, 69, 84, 93, 114,
      116, 117, 132, 142,
      144, 149, 150, 167–
      169, 176, 177, 197–200
Reye Syndrome, 173, 207
Rheumatism, 51, 55, 58, 61,
      69, 70, 78, 79, 85, 86,
      107, 114, 117, 120,
      125, 126, 172, 196, 206
Ringworm, 133, 168
Rosemary (*Rosmarinus
      officinalis*), 42, 193–
      194, 251
Rosemary House, 24
Rutin, 212, 228

Safety guidelines, 18–20, 46
Sage, 39, 42, 43, 261
Sage Mountain Herbal
      Products, 24
St. John's wort (*Hypericum
      perforatum*), 194–196,
      229, 240, 255, 261,
      268, 273, 275
St.-Mary's-thistle, 173
Salicin, 71–73, 171–172, 206,
      264
Salicin willow, 206
Salicylic acid, 212
Salt, 9, 28
Salves, 18

Saponins, 153

Saturated fat, 29

Saw palmetto (*Serenoa serrulata*), 38, 39, 196–198, 258, 268

Scabies, 56, 57

Scabwort, 115

School of Medical Herbalism, 20

Sciatica, 196

Scopoletin, 71

Scouring rush, 157

Selenium, 31, 159

Self-diagnosis, 20

Sexual vigor, 39, 104

Shave grass, 157

Sheep rot, 151

Shepherd's club, 176

Shingles, 81

Siberian ginseng (*Eleutherococcus senticosus*), 140, 141, 145–147, 258

Silica, 157, 158

Silymarin, 173

Simpler's joy, 204

Sinus problems, 88, 114

Skin care, 42–43, 51–52

Skin problems, 10, 53, 54, 92, 95, 114, 133, 134, 170

Slippery elm (*Ulmus rubra*), 32, 33, 198–199, 238

Smoking, 6, 8, 28, 29, 31–33, 36, 37, 40, 168, 169, 232, 243

Snakeweed, 68

Soldier's woundwort, 213

Sores, 48, 49, 80, 98, 127, 161

Sore throat, 17, 64, 65, 67, 127, 176, 177, 190, 198, 200, 213, 220, 269

Spleen, 65

Sprains, 168

Staunchgrass, 213

Sticklewort, 48

Stinkweed, 89

Stomach problems, 55, 57, 65, 73, 180, 186

Stress, 6–10, 32, 33, 40, 41, 84, 87, 141, 180, 195, 203, 205, 211, 212, 255, 269–270

Sugar, 9, 106

Sunburn, 11, 53, 195, 196, 271

Sundrops, 121

Sweating, 10, 74, 75

Sweet broom, 79

Sweet viburnum, 71

Swimming, 10

Swollen glands, 91, 177

Tachycardia, 175

Tannin, 206, 210, 212

Taylor's Herb Gardens, Inc., 24

Tea, 15–16, 18, 32, 34
Teething, 87
Tense constipation, 238
Tension, 9, 69, 87, 162–164, 180, 195, 203, 205
Testosterone, 104, 143
Thorny burr, 77
Thoroughwort, 74
Thousand seal, 213
Thrush, 275
Thujone, 213, 214
Thyme (*Thymus vulgaris*), 42, 199–201, 274
Thymol, 199
Tien Chi, 231
Tinctures, 14–15, 16
Tinnitus, 139
Tocopherol, 191
Tonics, 10, 27–29
Tonsillitis, 91, 112, 200, 209
Tooth and gum problems, 1, 67, 68, 90, 93, 178, 179, 190, 205, 209, 271
Torch, 176
Toxemia, 6
Trifolium, 191
Trigonelline, 50
Tuberculosis, 61, 112, 115

Ulcers, 80, 81, 165–166, 170, 182, 198, 208
Uric acid, 108
Urinary-tract infections, 28, 34–35, 48, 61, 65, 76, 91, 92, 101–102, 109, 157–159, 187, 201, 202, 220, 272
Ursolic acid, 201
Uva-ursi (*Arctostaphylos uva-ursi*), 76, 201–203, 272

Vaginal discharge, 49, 68, 102
Vaginal douches, 17–18
Valerian (*Valeriana officinalis*), 7, 41, 99, 175, 203–204, 224, 255, 259, 265, 266, 270
Valium, 203
Varicose veins, 67, 81, 86, 152, 156, 157, 170, 171, 195, 196, 210, 211, 214, 273
Vegetables, 8, 9, 30–33, 40, 243
Velvet dock, 115, 176
Venereal disease, 76
Verbena, 204
Vertigo, 139
Vervain (*Verbena officinalis*), 204–205, 232, 240, 270
Vitamin A, 105, 183
Vitamin B$_6$, 31, 40
Vitamin C, 31, 35, 50, 105, 183, 228, 234, 272
Vitamin D, 50
Vitamin E, 31, 50, 191, 234, 258, 275
Vitamin K, 50

Vitamins, 26
Vitex (*see* Agnus-castus)
Vomiting, 5, 10, 135, 136, 140, 169, 186

Walking, 10
Warts, 134
Water consumption, 9, 35
Water pennywort, 151
Water retention, 50, 79
Wax berry, 66
Wax myrtle, 66
Weight loss, 20
White willow (*Salix alba*), 206–207, 264, 265
Whooping cough, 57, 95, 115, 117, 132, 191, 192, 200, 274
Wild cherry bark (*Prunus serotina*), 208–209, 239, 240, 274
Wild indigo (*Baptisia tinctoria*), 209–210, 245
Wild sunflower, 115
Witch hazel (*Hamamelis virginiana*), 210–211, 253, 255, 273
Wolf's bane, 58

Wood betony (*Betonica officinalis*), 211–212, 219, 252
Wounds, 18, 67, 80, 81, 98, 113, 114, 127, 152, 170, 171, 178, 187, 190, 195, 196, 198, 205, 210–213, 274–275
Wrinkles, 114

Yarrow (*Achillea millefolium*), 49, 114, 212–214, 228, 231, 234, 247, 256, 269
Yeast infections (candidiasis), 18, 65, 113, 132, 184, 275–276
Yellow dock (*Rumex crispus*), 31, 34, 214–215, 221, 226, 230, 233, 237, 254, 260, 268, 273
Yellow root, 149
Yerba santa, 70
Yoga, 41
Yogurt, 35, 42
Yunnan Pai Yao, 274
Yuppie flu, 231

Zinc, 31